# A Guide to Aging

Published by :
**Lotus Press Publishers & Distributors**

# A Guide to Aging

**Prof. V.K. Ahluwalia**
Visiting Professor
Dr. B.R. Ambedkar Centre for Biomedical Research
University of Delhi, Delhi - 110 007, India.

**Dr. M. Ahluwalia**
Ex-CMO, WUS Health Center
University of Delhi, Delhi - 110 007, India

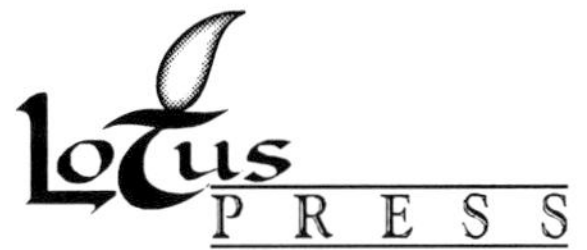


4735/22, Prakash Deep Building
Ansari Road, Darya Ganj,
New Delhi - 110002

**Lotus Press : Publishers & Distributors**
Unit No. 220, 2nd Floor, 4735/22, Prakash Deep Building,
Ansari Road, Darya Ganj, New Delhi- 110002
Ph.: 41325510, 98118-38000
• E-mail : lotuspress1984@gmail.com
www.lotuspress.co.in

**A Guide to Aging**



ISBN: 81-89093-95-9



*Printed & Published by* : **Lotus Press Publishers & Distributors,** New Delhi-02

# Preface

We have come across a large number of aged patients (senior citizens) who have a number of problems with their body and systems. Some of the common problems are dificulty in walking, wrinkles on the face, looking much older than their age and some medical problems. Their main concern is why they have aged so fast. The idea of writing this book originated by talking to the aged patients.

The present book deals with the effect of aging on various organs/parts of the body. An attempt has been made to explain how aging can be slowed down. However, being a natural phenomen, no one can prevent aging but the process can be considerably delayed. The factors that are responsible is to live healthy life in good surroundings, eat as for as possible, vegetables and fruits in their raw form or cooked lightly. One should take the food items so as to get the required vitamins, minerals and antioxidants which are essential to keep the body fit. One should avoid a stressful life and do a regular exercise programme. The suggestions given should be followed by all age group.

A very important aspect is to protect the body from life-robing diseases. Sime such diseases along with strategies to prevent them are discussed. It is hoped that the present book will be useful to all.

**Authors**

# Forward

Aging is a natural pheonenon that affects each and every part and systems of the body. This book on 'A Guide To Aging' written by Professor V.K. Ahluwalia and Dr. M. Ahluwalia, describes the effect of aging on various parts of the body.

Being a natural phenomenon, it is not possible to stop the aging process. However, the process can be considerable delayed. The authors have described the strategies for slowing down aging process. An important aspect is to protect the body from life robbing diseases along with strategies to prevent them have also been discussed. Some golden principles for delaying the onset of aging have also been included.

It is hoped that this book will be helpful to all ages of people, particularly the senior citizens.

**Dr. K.C. Goswami**
Chief Medical Officer
University of Delhi
Delhi - 110 007

# Contents

# 1

# INTRODUCTION

Aging is a natural phenomenon. Normally, anybody born in this world has to become an adult and finally become old before he dies. A person starts showing symptoms of aging anytime after 40-45 years of age. However, with the advancement of scientific procedures, it is now possible to considerably slow down the aging process (though it is not possible to stop it). For delaying aging, it is important to take a proper diet so that one gets reasonable amounts of Vitamins E, C, beta-carotene, Vitamins of the B group, minerals like chromium, zinc, calcium, magnesium, selenium, garlic, fruits, vegetables, soya beans, antioxidants etc. Each of these play an important role in slowing down the process of aging, keeping an individual's youth and vigor and stretching the life span.

Many scientists believe that aging is not an inevitable consequence of time. They consider it as a disease caused by a lifetime of environmental assaults to cells and this leads to a slow degeneration of the body resulting in breakdown of many of the body functions. ***There is evidence that one can interfere at any age with this deterioration.*** It is never too late to try to interrupt the process of aging.

# 2

# Effects of Aging

It is well known that aging affects each and every part and systems of the body. Some of the parts affected include the skin, face, hair, joints, nerve cells, heart, lungs, the digestive system, urinary bladder, kidneys, eyes, ears, taste buds, smell and the reproductive organs. A brief discussion of the effect of aging on all the above body parts and systems is given below.

## 2.1 The Skin

The most prominent effect of aging is the appearance of wrinkles and sagging of the skin. In fact the function of the skin is to withstand the pressures of moving limbs, internal movement of blood vessels and muscles. With age, skin loses its flexibility, which results in wrinkles, sags and loss of firmness. In fact all parts of the skin, viz., the epidermis, the dermis, oil glands and fat tissues are affected by aging. The cells in the epidermis (the outer layer of the skin) are depleted more quickly than they are replaced. This results in thinning of this layer leading to formation of wrinkles. The dermis is located immediately beneath the epidermis. The dermis contains many molecules, which keep the skin in form and maintain its structure. With age, cross-links occur with greater frequency in the collagen protein resulting in loss of flexibility. The sweat glands, located within the dermis play a vital role in regulating the body temperature. With aging, our ability to adapt to temperature changes is reduced. This is attributed to decreased secretion of fluid by the sweat glands. Finally, the fat cells are present as an even blanket beneath the dermis. With age, the layers of fat cells become thinner, leaving irregular 'clumps' of fatty deposits.

## 2.2 The Face

The aging process affects all the three layers of the human skin (discussed above). Fig. 2.1 illustrates the affects of aging on the face after the age of 60.

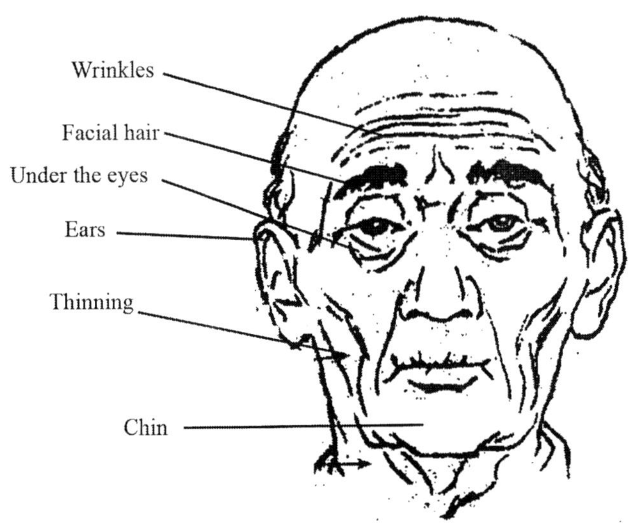


**Fig. 2.1. Effects of aging on face**

As seen in Fig. 2.1, the skin wrinkles due to thinning of epidermis. Due to aging, one generally loses the hair on scalp (alternatively there is thinning of hair on the scalp) and the eyebrows of men get thicker, and hair begin to sprout on the inner canal of the outer ear. The postmenopausal women, due to depletion of hormones can grow facial hair, especially on the chin.

With aging, bags under the eyes occur due to accumulation of fluids under the eyes. The appearance of a dark pigment below the eyes give an appearance of 'sunken eyes'. The ears and the nose tend to broaden and become longer, later in life. The face becomes thin, the skin appears as if there are no teeth in the mouth. Finally, the skin below the chin sags with aging, also known as double chin.

## 2.3 The Hair

The aging process affects groups of cells within the hair follicle, where the germ centers (where a group of cells manufacture hair shaft proteins) and melanocytes (another group of cells which manufacture the proteins involved in hair color) exist. We, generally notice that the hair turn gray as we age. In fact, in the aging process hair turn white. This happens due to selective and progressive deactivation of melanocytes. The gray color, which we see, is a mixture of the original color and white. Hair loss (or getting bald) occurs because the cells that manufacture hair protein, the germ centers are selectively destroyed or deactivated. When the original hair shed, no replacement occurs. Depending on the degree or amount of hair loss, there may be either thinning of hair on the scalp or complete baldness.

## 2.4 The Joints

As we age, our joints become less flexible. A synovial joint (named for the characteristic presence of a fluid called, synovial fluid) is shown in Fig. 2.2. As aging occurs, the tissues within the joint begin to break down. The joints become less flexible due to the combined deterioration of tendons, ligaments and cartilage. Though the deterioration is attributed to aging, these can also occur any time during adulthood.

The synovial fluid (not available in all joints) gives cushion to the forces of movement between the bones. With age, the synovial fluid gets thinner and affects the flexibility of the joint.

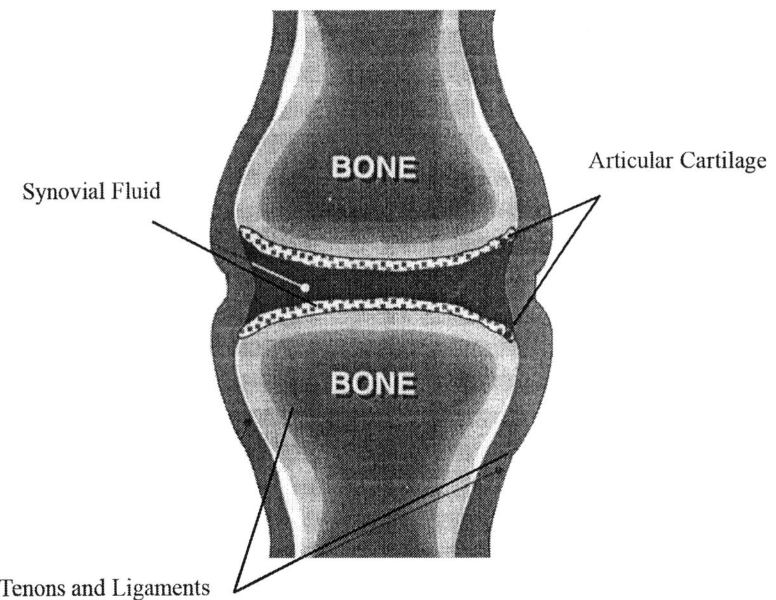


**Fig. 2.2. Effect of aging on joints**

The articular cartilage (Fig. 2.2) normally provides a protective coating against friction from bones rubbing against each other. With age, the cartilage becomes opaque, cracks and frays; these changes result in increased joint pain and decreased mobility.

With age, changes in collagen and elastic production occur in tendons and ligaments, resulting in fragmented tissues and so the new structures become less resilient with increasing loss of flexion and extension. Calcification also occurs due to age related injury.

With advancing age, the joints are subjected to extreme daily trauma resulting in cumulative injuries. The elastic and resilient original tissues are replaced by fibrous and calcified new material; this results in achiness, stiffness and a reduction in effective movement.

## 2.5 The Nerve Cells

With aging a number of nerve cells in the brain are lost. The nerve cells suffer neural loss. After the age of 60, the percentage of cells remaining in Occipital lobe, locus coeruleus, purkinje fibers and thalamus (Fig. 2.3) are 50,60,75 and 100% compared to the number of cells at a younger stage.

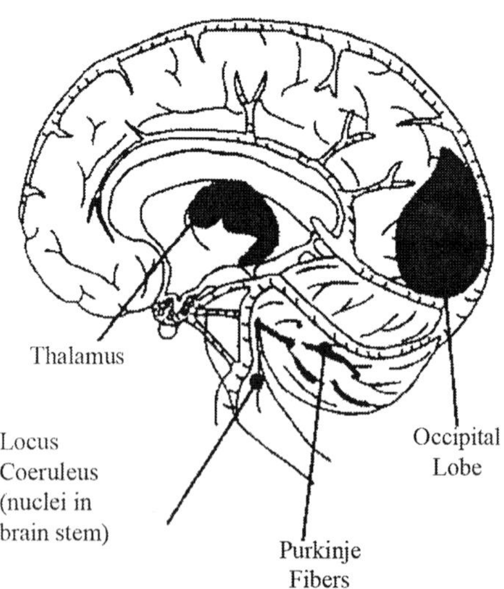


**Fig. 2.3. Nerve cell centers in the brain**

As seen, the nerve cells in thalamus do not exhibit any appreciable loss.

## 2.6 The Heart

As we age, the walls around the left vertical (Fig. 2.4) thicken. The enlargement reduces the ability of the heart to pump large volume of blood to the body. As a result the following cardiac functions decline.

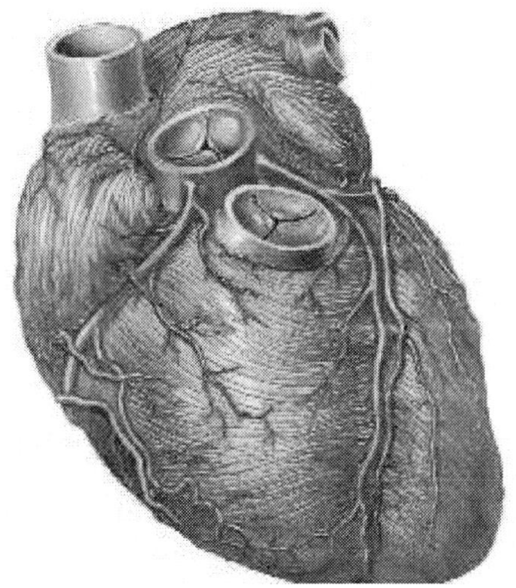

**Fig. 2.4. The Heart and its parts**

### Decrease in stroke volume

Stroke volume is the amount of blood the heart can pump at each beat. With aging, the stroke volume decreases, as less blood goes through.

### Decrease in cardiac output

Cardiac output is the stroke volume multiplied by the pulse per minute. With aging, the stroke volume decreases, thereby reducing the total cardiac output per unit time.

**Decline in oxygen consumption**

The consumption of oxygen is calculated by multiplying the oxygen extracted from blood by the cardiac output. So as the output declines and the ability of tissues to be fed also declines.

## 2.7 The Lungs

The breathing occurs because the muscles in our chest expand the volume of the lungs, creating a partial vacuum. As a result of this expansion, air flows in (inhalation)(Fig. 2.5(a)). During exhalation (Fig. 2.5(b)) it is important to evacuate as much air from the lungs as possible; this results in more efficient flushing of waste products. In addition, it also creates more room for fresh air to be delivered to the blood.

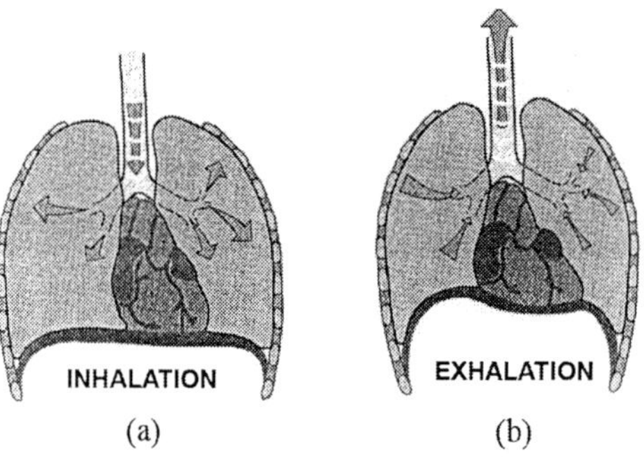


**Fig. 2.5. Lungs depicting (a) inhalation (b) Exhalation**

During breathing there is an exchange of molecules. The red blood cells, laden with carbon dioxide arrive at the alveoli. The carbon dioxide diffuses from the red blood cells and is exhaled from the body. The oxygen diffuses from the alveoli and enters the red blood cells, which transport it throughout the body.

As we age, it is increasingly difficult to get the old air out. This in turn makes it increasingly difficult to oxygenate blood. This creates a disastrous situation. The old air already has a lot of its oxygen taken out from it by the blood cells. Also, the old air is filled with waste products. The overall effect is a reduced level of oxygen in the blood. This results in a type of starvation for the tissues. So for older people, it is difficult to perform as much physical activity as younger people.

In view of the above, it can be said that it is the fault of the lungs that blood gets less oxygen with increasing age.

### 2.8 The Digestive System

The major organs involving the digestive system are affected to different degree as we age. Some organs exhibit no loss of function while others show changes. Following are given the changes effected in some of the major organs of the digestive system as we age.

***Saliva:***

The parotid glands secrete less saliva as we age. This results in discomfort in talking, chewing and dryness in the mouth.

***Swallowing:***

The muscles, which are responsible for swallowing, weaken. However, there is no significant loss of function.

***Stomach:***

The muscles of the stomach become weak with age and the content of the gastric juice becomes less. There is, however, no change in the function.

*Liver:*

In liver also, there is no functional change, though there are some alterations in the overall architecture of various tissues of the liver.

*Pancreas:*

There is a reduction in the fat-eating molecules secreted into the intestine. The liver can adequately compensate this loss.

*Large intestine:*

There is no loss of function though there is reduction in lubricating mucus and a weakening of the muscles, which push the waste into the rectum.

*Small Intestine:*

The small intestine helps in absorbing nutrients from the digested food and tossing them to the blood stream. As we age, the ability to absorb specific molecules decreases. Thus, calcium is not fully absorbed. However, this has been attributed to a decline in Vitamin D levels. Two other vitamins, viz., Vitamin B12 and folic acid are not fully absorbed by small intestines.

## 2.9 The Bladder and the Kidney

As we age, our ability to hold urine and clean blood changes. This is due to changes in the structure of the bladder and the kidney; this in turn affects the life style and health.

With age, the connective tissue and muscles (which are responsible for the expansion and contraction of the bladder) of the bladder weaken (Fig. 2.6(a)) resulting in an overall decrease in our ability to store urine. It also reduces the efficiency of emptying the bladder when urinating.

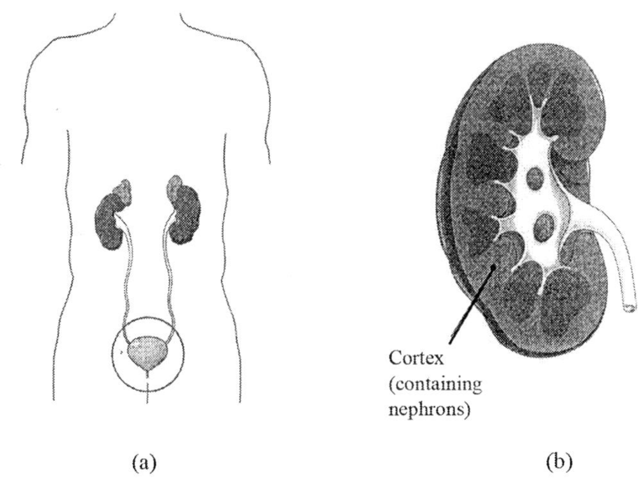


**Fig. 2.6 (a) Bladder and (b) Kidney**

The kidney shrinks as we age. Their appearance becomes smoother, reducing the aggregate surface for filtering. These changes reflect alteration occurring within the nephrons (composed of blood vessels). The blood is filtered here. The nephrons are located in the cortex of the human kidney (Fig. 2.6(b)). As we age, there is a marked reduction in the cleaning of impurities from blood.

## 2.10 The Eyes

The tissues in eyes are affected as we age. Eyes in an organized form collect the light so that the brain can interpret what is seen. Light rays travel through the cornea and enter the pupil, a hole in the eye whose diameter is controlled by tiny muscles in the iris. (Fig. 2.7)

The light enters the lens through the pupil, and focuses it to the back of the eyeball. To perform this task, the lens must be able to stretch and expand; this is controlled by muscle structures collectively known as ciliary body. From the back of the eye, the light is met by nerves that make the retina. The specific neurons in the retina capture the light and respond to various characteristics including wavelengths of the received light. Once stimulated, the signal is sent through the optic nerve to the brain. The brain organizes and helps to interpret this input, allowing us to 'see'. All this implies that we really see with our brains.

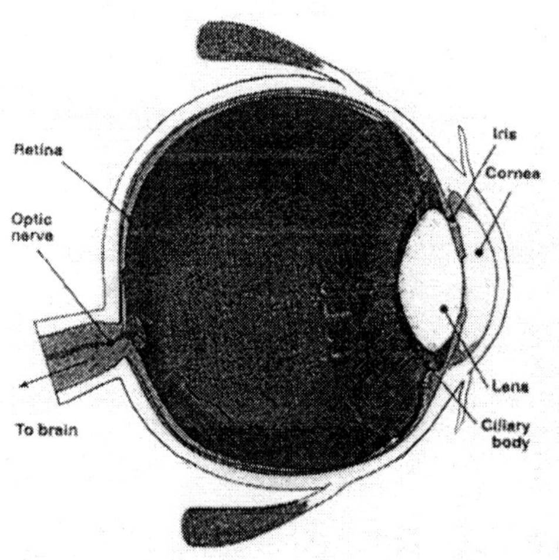


**Fig. 2.7. Eyes and its various parts**

The aging process greatly affects our eyes, changing the way we see the world. New layers of tissues are added to the lens with increasing age. The older tissues are not removed. This results in thickening of the lens with age, squeezing the older layer in the middle. This change causes far sightedness. The ciliary body, the muscles, vessels and the connective tissues also age with time. As the muscles atrophy, the ability to focus light rays back to the eye is diminished.

The structure and internal composition of the cornea also changes with age. The cornea flattens with passing years. Thus, the consequent change in visual field often requires using corrective lens. The muscles in the iris atrophy with age. The pupil becomes more restricted in size. This requires additional light to see objects within the visual field. The atrophy also reduces the flexibility of the iris. This implies that we do not respond as quickly to changes in environmental light.

With age, the color of the lens of the eye becomes gradually yellow and we are not able to discriminate between green, blue and violet wavelength of light. This is because as we age, changes in the lens cause less light to reach the specialized cells, which helps us differentiate between colors.

## 2.11 The Ears

Aging affects all three parts of ears, altering the way we hear. We possess outer, middle and an inner ear. The sound waves first enter the outer ear through a large external flap called the pinna (Fig. 2.8). The wave travels through the external auditory/ canal until it reaches the eardrum. When the sound wave touches the drum, the ensuing vibrations rattle the three bones (called the malleus, incus and stapes) of the middle ear. The third bone (stapes) is attached to a part of the inner ear known as the vestibule. (Fig. 2.8). The inner ear is a complex structure filled with fluid and nerves. As the staples vibrate, a sloshing motion is produced. This motion is registered by the nerves, which send signals to the brain. This is how sound is heard.

As we age, the pinna begins to drop due to changes in certain proteins. Hair grows on the external auditory gland.

The canal also gets dry due to a loss of sweat glands. This results in building up earwax, which severely affect hearing.

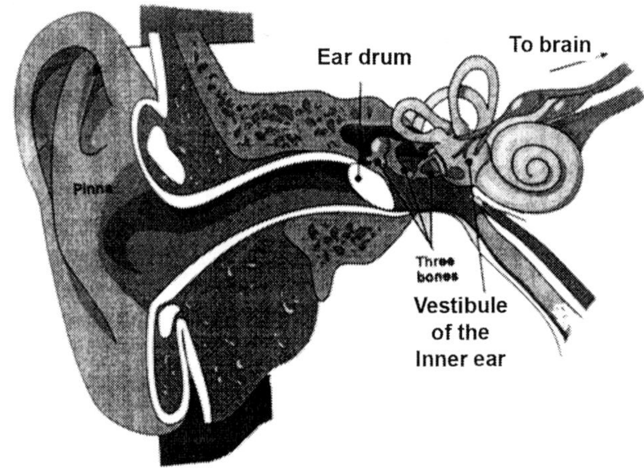


**Fig. 2.8. Ear and its parts**

The eardrum becomes thinner and more flaccid with age. Atrophy occurs in the muscles, which support the membrane. Due to this, the eardrum is less easily vibrated by sound waves. The joints on the three bones also degenerate with time. Ligaments and muscles (which connect the bones) follow the normal aging process. With age, calcification occurs between the bones, with the result that the vibrations from the eardrum are not transferred efficiently to the inner ear. Also, the blood supply that nourishes the tissues in the inner ear decreases. The nerves that sense and conduct signals to the brain die and are not replaced. Even excess bone formation occurs. All these factors result in hearing defect known as presbycusis.

As we age, the ability to hear the frequencies of human voice is generally retained. However, the ability to hear some specific frequencies of sound is lost.

## 2.12 The Taste

Aging changes the ability to taste. In fact, we experience taste through a collection of cells connected to a nerve. This structure is called a taste bud. Various regions of the tongue are responsible for specific tastes. (Fig. 2.9)

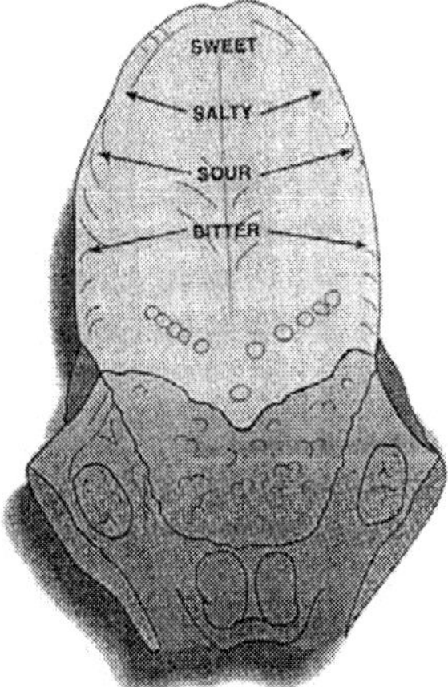


**Fig. 2.9. Tongue and regions of specific tastes**

Flavours are experienced because a molecule of food lands on the receptors on the taste bud's surface. This excites the nerve beneath; subsequently the signal is shifted to the brain.

We lose our sense of flavor with age only gradually; there is equal reduction in all areas.

## 2.13 The Smell

The sense of smell is intimately connected to our ability to taste. The organs that mediate our sense of smell are the olfactory bulb, tracks and nerves in the upper respiratory system. (Fig. 2.10) They are located on the ceiling of the cavity as shown in Fig 2.10. The cells in the olfactory bulb possess receptors on their surface. When an odor - bearing molecule binds to a receptor, the olfactory nerve gets stimulated; the signal goes to the brain and smell is registered.

Till about the age of 65, our ability to differentiate odors remains more or less constant. After 65, there is some loss. The amount of reduction varies between individuals.

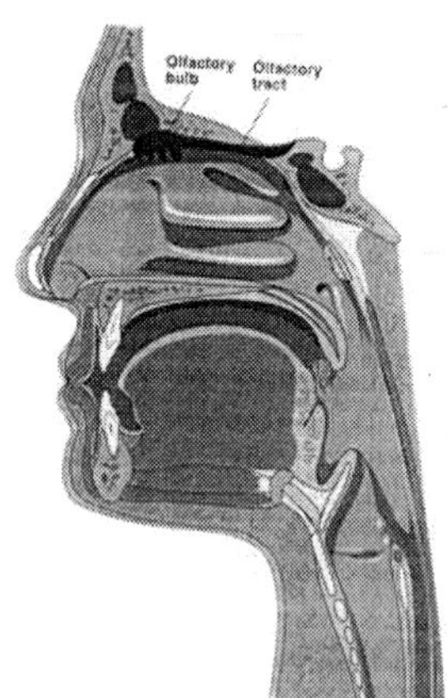


**Fig. 2.10.**

The difference in the ability of individuals is that environmental pollution may play a role in affecting the integrity of the olfactory system.

## 2.14 The Reproductive System

We now know how aging affects various parts of the body. In fact, aging also affects our reproductive system. However in terms of enjoyment such changes mean nothing. Women and men age very differently with respect to sexual behavior. In women, after menopause, the hormone estrogen is not produced (or produced in very small amount). In fact, estrogen is responsible for maintenance of all female reproductive structures including development of breasts and development of the secondary sexual characteristics. So with age, women have menopause and all the functions which estrogen does, are hindered to a great extent. After menopause, the breasts are affected. Throughout the body, subcutaneous fat begins to accumulate especially near the waist, which creates uneven bulges.

The aging of men's reproductive organs is much less pronounced. There is gradual tapering off of reproductive viability compared to women whose reproductive viability virtually ceases after menopause. Men can continue to father children even after 60 years of age. However, the time needed to obtain an erection after stimulation is 3-4 times more than in younger people. Older people take more time for ejaculation.

# 3

# WHY WE AGE? WHAT CAUSES IT?

Like death, aging is universal. The question is how rapidly one ages. The individual life span to a major extent depends on an individual. For a long time, scientists have been trying to find ways to expand mortality and avoid the curse of old age so that we can live at our fullest capacity until the end of our life.

The secrets of aging lie in individual cells. A number of theories have been put forward. It is believed that a major part of aging is explained by the free radical theory of aging. According to this theory, chemical particles called free radicals damage the cells. Thin cellular damage accumulates over the years, until one reaches a point of no return. Free radicals are regarded as chemical substances that contain an odd number of electrons. These are made in our bodies all the times, and if they are not destroyed, cells can be damaged. In fact, free radicals can also lead to the development of cancer. The formation of free radicals can be visualized as follows: when high energy in any form (light radiation) hits an atom, an electron is kicked out of the orbit. All the energy that forces the electron of the orbit, is transferred directly to the electron, making it highly energetic and unstable. The high-energy electron goes into another atom, making it extremely unstable. This high-energy atom with its extra electron is called a free radical. (Fig. 3.1)

The unstable free radical must get rid of all the extra energy for the atom to become stable again. So the radical transfers its energy to nearby substances. All these reactions take place within a fraction of second. Once free radicals are made in the body, the high energy is transferred to the body tissues particularly to the polysaturated fats found in the cell membranes. Therefore, if one eats unsaturated fats, more free radicals are absorbed by the cell membranes and the risk is higher for the membrane disrupted by the free radicals. If free radicals are not counteracted, this process can lead to the development of cancer tissues. In other words, the free radicals damage the cells.

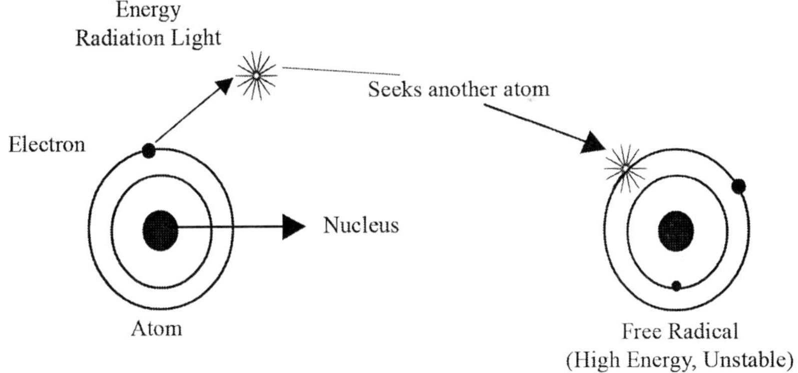


**Fig. 3.1. Formation of free radical**

In the body, free radicals are formed by oxygen, which is a very important constituent of the air we inhale. Under certain circumstances, oxygen can be activated or split with high energy into damaging radicals (super oxide) or a high energy, unstable non-radical called singlet oxygen. The latter is very unstable having high energy and is very destructive to normal body cells and tissues. Under different circumstances, oxygen radicals can be both beneficial and harmful to the human body. The beneficial application is when a phagocyte kills invading bacteria. This destruction is accomplished by oxygen radicals, which are made by the phagocyte when a foreign substance like bacterium invades and is taken inside the phagocyte. Alternatively, oxygen radicals can produce hydro peroxides, which damage cell membranes, thereby altering the cell function. This can lead to malfunctioning of the cells including development of cancer. Singlet oxygen, a very high-energy form of oxygen has a shorter life than oxygen radical but damages cells and tissues quickly.

As already stated, the free radicals can be neutralized by antioxidants, the compounds that give up on their electrons thus returning the free radicals to normal state and stopping their destructive capability. In the body there is an inbuilt arsenal of defenses, made up of enzymes and other chemicals called antioxidants. These agents stop the formation of free radicals and also repair the damage caused by free radicals. Even after these, the inbuilt defense mechanism is not able to look after all the free radicals. It is the accumulation of cellular damage and the rubbish from incomplete repair that fuels the aging process. It is believed that at the age of about 50, 20-25% of cellular protein turns into junk by free radical attacks. The free radicals attack the fatty molecules, leaving it spoiled, just as butter out of the refrigerator becomes rancid. In a way, it can be said that as we age, we chemically resemble a piece of meat that has been left for long in the open air and sun.

# 4

# Why Can't We Live Forever?

It is the law of nature that everybody who comes into this world ultimately ages. In fact, nature builds up this into our genes. However, nature cares about us only till 40-50 years of age when we have performed our duties of reproduction. In the natural process, as we get older, two important process hasten aging. The first factor is the rate of increase of cell damaging free radical reactions. The second factor is our inborn ability to neutralize the free radicals and repair the damage from free radicals loses vigor as we age. This implies that the older we get, the more damage accumulates in our cells and the aging process speeds up. Thus, as we get older or as we age the inbuilt defense against free radicals decreases. Ultimately, we all lose the battle of life to one thing or the other. It is only a matter of chance how life is terminated. If one does not die, for example of cancer, one may soon die of some other rapidly developing disease, for example of the cardiovascular system.

To sum up, we can say that aging is a disease. The life span of a human being reflects the level of free radical damage that accumulates, cells just cannot survive properly anymore and then give up.

# 5

# Slowing Down Aging

It is for sure that nobody can live forever, since we cannot stop aging. However, the aging process can be considerably slowed down. Checking or neutralizing the free radicals and or repairing the damage caused by free radicals can help achieve this. Thus what is needed is a delicate balance - enough antioxidants to keep the free radicals under control so that they cannot overrun the body causing havoc. The presence of outside antioxidants is essential particularly when the internal mechanism of the body is not able to deal with free radicals and their effects. When there are more free radicals than antioxidants, there is a problem in the system. This imbalance damages the cells resulting in accumulated damage. The antiaging antioxidants can be built up in the system by the following:

- Eat plenty of antioxidants; the big three powerful antioxidants are Vitamin E, beta-carotene, and Vitamin C. Also antioxidants are present in herbs and foods such as garlic, broccoli, tea and tomatoes. These antioxidants flood the blood stream and hence the cells with neutralizers of free radicals.
- Take supplements, herbs, vitamins and other food constituents that stimulate the enzymes to rev up the body's detoxification system that zap free

radicals. Broccoli is good; it contains sulforaphane, which stimulates mechanism that neutralize the free radicals.

- Do not take foods that are easily oxidized and generate free radicals inside the cell. Some examples are corn oil and sunflower oil, margarine and dried eggs, which are used, in a number of processed foods.

Thus, by consuming antioxidants, people will be able to live longer.

## 5.1 Free Radicals Versus Antioxidants

We can take quantum leaps in our ability to combat aging if we understand that,

- Free radicals damage cells, causing aging
- Antioxidants block free radical damage
- So antioxidants help combat aging.

Once we have understood the above three basics to prevent aging, the rest is obvious. Try to find antioxidants, use them and thus slow down aging, stay younger and live longer.

There are more anti-aging agents in the universe than one could imagine, some of these are in the form of vitamins, minerals, natural enzymes, amino acids, herbs, plants, foods and other natural substances.

A number of studies conducted in institutions such as Harvard, University of California, Tufts, John Hopkins, Stanford, Yale and others have proved that anti-aging agents have antioxidant activity that delay the aging process by warding off free radical damage to cells. Many antioxidant substances like Vitamin E and Vitamin C as well as coenzyme Q-10 may all work individually and together to prevent the process of aging, prevent cancer, heart disease and brain degeneration. It has been recognized that deficiency of these substances (or antioxidants) generates our epidemic of premature and needless aging.

Vitamins and minerals are needed while aging. These save the arteries from destruction, the brain from damage, cells from cancer and immune system from degenerating. In fact, both vitamins and minerals slow down some of the consequences of growing old. It has been shown that not taking vitamins and minerals is an invitation to reckless aging and premature death.

### 5.1.1 Vitamins

Antioxidants such as Vitamin C, Vitamin E and beta-carotene may prove as potent as antibiotics and vaccines in fighting diseases. A number of studies have shown that people who take vitamins delay the onset or the severity of aging diseases. It has been found that:

- People who take vitamins, especially Vitamin C and Vitamin E, live several years longer than people who do not.
- Vitamins (sometimes a simple multi vitamin pill) rejuvenate the faltering immune system as one ages.
- Heart disease victims have low blood and tissue levels of dietary antioxidants including Vitamin E, Vitamin C and beta-carotene. Even people susceptible to cancer also have low blood and tissue levels of Vitamin C, Vitamin E, beta-carotene and selenium.

- A deficiency of Vitamin B group can trigger senility, artery damage, heart attack and some cancers. Taking these vitamins often prevents or remedies these problems.
- Even a marginal chromium deficiency can precipitate a midlife slide into diabetes and cardiovascular disease.
- Calcium and Vitamin D supplements after a year can dramatically prevent broken bones even in eight-year-old kids.
- Regular vitamin takers have about 25% lower risk of developing cataracts and reduce considerably (about 60-70%) the risk of common skin cancer.

The belief that the natural foods can give everything you need to get through the tough years of old age, is not exactly true particularly due to the hazards of modern civilization including polluted environment, pesticides, radiation from nuclear energy, auto exhaust, smog, fat and chemically loaded processed food all of which set up the free radical attacks on the human body causing aging prematurely. It is recommended that one should take the following daily to avoid aging.

| | |
|---|---|
| Vitamin E | 400 iu |
| Vitamin C | 500 mg |
| Beta-carotene | 25,000 iu |

One should understand that vitamin supplements work in the same way as wearing a seat belt, which does not give a license to drive recklessly, but just protects in case of an accident. Similarly, vitamin supplements do not give a license to eat poorly and otherwise abuse one's health, but provide an additional cushion of protection.

Following are given some special points one should know about vitamins to fend off aging.

- It is not correct to think that food can give all the vitamins and minerals one needs to slow down the process of aging.
- To slow down aging, it is necessary to take mega doses of antioxidant vitamins and minerals. Notably vitamins are Vitamin E, Vitamin C and beta-carotene.
- Aging and its consequences are partly a vitamin-mineral 'deficiency disease'.
- Vitamins and minerals also help to fight the chronic age-driven epidemic of heart disease and cancer.
- The main way vitamins and minerals combat aging is by boosting antioxidant activity, helping neutralize the free radicals that are the prime cause of aging.
- Contrary to one's fear vitamins and minerals in antiaging doses are safe and free of side affects.
- Numerous vitamins and minerals work together to protect against aging. It has been shown that antioxidants work better in combination than individually.

There are a number of advantages to people who take antioxidants. Some of these are:

- A number of studies show that the death rate is down to 50% from any cause in people taking both Vitamin C and Vitamin E. Research indicates that elderly vitamin takers have only one third as many heart disease death as non-vitamin takers.
- Taking antioxidant vitamins cuts down cancer

deaths by 10-12%, presumably the antioxidants worked by guarding cells from free radical damage. Experts recommend a daily dose of 15 mg of beta-carotene, 30 mg of Vitamin E and 50 micrograms of selenium. The mega doses of vitamins also help fight existing cancer cases.

- Taking 50 mg of beta-carotene daily for long term (2-4 years) by people suffering from angina (chest pain) reduced the heart attacks or strokes by about 50%.
- Taking a simple one a day multivitamin pill boosts immune system significantly in older people with good diets.
- Men taking a multi-vitamin pill a day are only 70% as likely to develop cataracts as non-vitamin takers.

### 5.1.1.1 Vitamin E

It is known to stop aging, if one does not take any other vitamins, Vitamin E should be taken. It is virtually impossible to get Vitamin E from food to fight diseases like cancer and heart disease and get immunity to diseases unless one eats more than 500 calories a day, most of them in fats. Therefore Vitamin E supplements are necessary to combat aging problems. Some of the benefits of taking Vitamin E supplements include:

- Vitamin E blocks artery clogging. In fact, it fights our greatest aging factor arthersclerosis (the gradual clogging and hardening of the arteries).
- It dramatically reduces the appearance of heart disease.

- It rejuvenates old arteries.
- It rejuvenates immunity.
- It thwarts cancer.
- It relieves arthritis.
- It postpones cataracts. In fact, it arrests and even reverses the development of cataracts.
- It retards overall brain and blood aging.

Vitamin E is a fat-soluble antioxidant and so it best works in the fattiest parts of the system. It appears especially critical in preventing brain, artery and immune system deterioration because the brain and immune cell membranes are fatty and arteries are very susceptible to damage from fat. In fact, it can be said that Vitamin E acts as a fire extinguisher to destroy free radicals and so prevent free radicals that turn fat in the brain and blood rancid, disturbing normal functioning and making the tissues age faster.

Experts consider a daily dose of 400-800 iu very safe with no known side effects. However, Vitamin E like aspirin has mild anticoagulant activity, 'thinning of blood' and is not recommended to people taking anticoagulant drugs or facing surgery. Taking mega doses (about 3200 iu daily) may have some toxic affects; signs include headaches, diarrhea, and elevated blood pressure. If one is taking anticoagulants or suspects any type of bleeding problems, it is advised to consult a doctor before taking Vitamin E.

#### 5.1.1.2 Vitamin C

It stops aging and prolongs life. *Linus Pauling*, two-time noble prizewinner died of cancer at the age of 93.

Just before his death he said, 'I attribute my health largely to the intake of Vitamin C and minerals.' Although he died of cancer, he believed that Vitamins had delayed the onset of cancer by about 20 years. He claimed to have had no cold since he began taking high doses of Vitamin C. Following are given some of the benefits of taking Vitamin C.

- Vitamin C immunizes against cancer.
- It saves arteries. It offers wholesale protection to arteries. It reduces bad type LDL cholesterol that destroys arteries. Vitamin C lowers high blood pressure and strengthens blood vessel walls.
- It raises immunity and boosts the immune function.
- Vitamin C reverses aging by rejuvenating white blood cells in elderly people.
- It improves sperms and restores male fertility. Studies have shown that it heals sperm and prevents male induced birth defects in non-smoking men.
- Vitamin C prevents lung disease like chronic bronchitis or asthma.
- It combats gum diseases like bleeding gums, deep pockets and receding gums.
- It prevents cataracts.

Vitamin C is a water-soluble antioxidant that traps and neutralizes free radicals in the watery part of the tissues. It also regenerates exhausted Vitamin E and spurns enzymes to search and destroy free radicals. Since the body does not store water soluble Vitamin C, one must eat it regularly to keep the cells supplied.

Unlike Vitamin E, Vitamin C is plentiful in food supply. So the best course is to eat plenty of Vitamin C - rich fruits and vegetables. However, to be safe one should take a Vitamin C supplement in addition to, not as a substitute for fruits and vegetables. One should also remember that fruits and vegetables also contain other antioxidants, which are necessary for delaying aging. Foods high in Vitamin C are sweet pepper, cantaloupe, papaya, strawberries, brussels, sprouts, citrus fruits, juices, kiwi fruit, broccoli and tomatoes. Taking Vitamin C is a type of insurance against aging.

Following are given some of the benefits of taking Vitamin C for slowing down aging and increasing the life span.

- Vitamin C suppresses high blood pressure
- It raises good type HDL-cholesterol
- It boosts levels of the body's most potent free radical enemy - glutathione.
- It inhibits bad type LDL cholesterol from becoming toxic (rancid or oxidized) and able to clog arteries.
- It prevents fatty deposits from artery walls.
- It reduces chances of heart attack.
- It improves immune functioning.
- It cuts odds of asthma, chronic bronchitis and other lung and breathing problems.
- It prevents oxidative damage to eyes warding off cataracts and other age related eye diseases.
- It protects sperm from free radical damage causing birth defects.
- It restores fertility in men.
- It fights cancer by thwarting formation of carcinogens, blocking free radical DNA damage

(a first step to cancer), prevents genes and viruses from switching on cancer activity, regulating immunity and slowing tumor growth.

It is believed by the experts that a daily 250-1000 mg is adequate to take care of ordinary ravages of aging and age related diseases. However, many scientists believe that several hundred thousand mg (about 2000-3000 mg) of Vitamin C give additional antiaging benefits.

Vitamin C is very safe. However, taking 'too much' may cause diarrhea, nausea and heartburn in some persons. To keep your cells on total antioxidant alert with Vitamin C, one should take supplements quota 3 or 4 times a day rather than one big dose, since in one time daily, the body eliminates large doses of Vitamin C (being water soluble).

### 5.1.1.3 Beta-carotene

It is considered to be an extra antiaging insurance. We have now known that taking both Vitamin E and Vitamin C help to save from aging. However, maximum aging slowdown can be possible if in addition to Vitamin E and C, lots of beta-carotene—from fruits and vegetables and/or pills is taken. Beta-carotene, the yellow pigment of carrots has extra antioxidant powers. Beta-carotene in short prevents overall bodily deterioration. A special advantage of taking beta-carotene is that it has additional antiaging powers. In the body, beta-carotene is in Vitamin A, which has antiaging qualities of its own, especially in bolstering immunity. Some of the ways in which beta-carotene can fight aging is given below:

- **Beta-carotene blocks cancer.** In fact, it is one antioxidant, which should be invariably taken if one wants to avoid cancer. Studies have shown that people taking high doses of beta-carotene in their diet are about half as likely to develop cancers notably of the lung, mouth, throat, esophagus, larynx, stomach and bladder. Some other studies have shown that beta-carotene blocks the development of cancer of the cervix and colon cancer in men. In fact, beta-carotene is believed to be a cancer chemo-preventing agent. It blocks the proliferation of cancer cells. It should be understood that the effects caused by longtime cigarette smoking (the cause of cancer of the lungs) can not be neutralized by beta-carotene in a short span of time. It takes about 10-12 years of high doses of beta-carotene to thwart the onset of cancer.

- **Beta-carotene prevents heart attacks.** It keeps the arteries from clogging and thus wards off cardiovascular diseases. This protection comes only after about two years of taking beta-carotene. It is recommended (the alliance for aging research, Washington) that adults should take 10 mg (17,000 iu) to 30 mg (50,000 iu) of beta-carotene daily.
- **Prevents stroke.** Stroke, the most feared consequence of aging can be prevented (or chances of stroke considerably reduced) by taking beta-carotene. One should consume lots of beta-carotene packed carrots and spinach to reduce the risk of stroke.
- **Beta-carotene stimulates immune functioning.** A number of studies have shown that older men and women who took 30-60 mg beta-carotene daily for 2 months had more natural killer cells, T-helper

cells and activated lymphocytes. Such immune cells help protect the body from cancer and viral and bacterial infections. Natural killer cells are particularly important in fighting cancer and taking 50 mg of beta-carotene every day significantly raises natural killer cells in the blood.

One can get lots of beta-carotene in fruits and vegetables (Table 5.1). The vegetables should be lightly cooked; heavy cooking destroys beta-carotene.

**Table 5.1. Foods containing beta-carotene**

| **Food** | **Amount of beta-carotene (mg)** |
|---|---|
| Carrot juice (1 cup) | 24.2 |
| Sweet potato (1 medium) | 10.0 |
| Apricots dried (10 halves) | 6.2 |
| Carrot, raw (1 medium) | 5.7 |
| Spinach, cooked (½ cup) | 4.9 |
| Cantaloupe (1/8) | 4.0 |
| Turnip green, cooked (½ cup) | 3.9 |
| Pumpkin, cooked (½ cup) | 3.7 |
| Apricots, fresh (2) | 2.5 |
| Spinach, raw (1 cup) | 2.3 |
| Tomato juice (1 cup) | 2.2 |
| Spaghetti squash, cooked (½ cup) | 1.9 |
| Mustard green, cooked (½ cup) | 1.9 |
| Beet green, cooked (½ cup) | 1.8 |
| Grapefruit, pink or red (½ cup) | 1.6 |
| Mango (½) | 1.4 |
| Bell peppers, sweet red (½ cup) | 1.1 |
| Romaine lettuce, raw (1 cup) | 1.1 |
| Watermelon (1 slice) | 1.1 |
| Broccoli, cooked (½ cup) | 1.0 |

For extra insurance against aging, a supplement of 10-15 mg of beta-carotene a day is recommended by the experts. Beta-carotene should be taken with meals because some fat in the diet is necessary for its absorption. Without a little fat, beta-carotene pills are a waste. On the basis of number of studies it has been found that taking divided doses of beta-carotene thrice a day with meal, boosts blood concentration of the vitamin three times higher than taking a single total dose once a day. One should make sure that the supplement is of beta-carotene and not just Vitamin A, which can be toxic.

Some of the antiaging effects of beta-carotene are given below:

- It prevents cancers particularly of lung, stomach and breast.
- Prevents stroke.
- Prevents heart attacks.
- Prevents clogging of arteries by blocking oxidation of cholesterol.
- Destroys tumor cells.
- Stimulates immune functions.
- Prevents cataract.
- Causes lesions in the mouth to disappear or regress.

Beta-carotene is one of the most non-toxic vitamins. A daily dose of 10-30 mg (17,000 to 50,000 iu) has been recommended by experts.

All the three-antioxidant vitamins, viz., Vitamin E, Vitamin C and beta-carotene fight aging better when taken together than one or two alone.

### 5.1.1.4 The B-group vitamins

The B Vitamins are another group of anti-aging vitamins. These vitamins delay aging by taking care of the heart and the mental faculties as one grows old. In fact, one needs all the vitamins of group B (commonly called the B Vitamin) to delay aging, but three of these viz., Vitamin B12, B6 and folic acid are most important due to their antiaging powers.

#### 5.1.1.4.1 Vitamin B12

Vitamin B12 is essential for proper mental functioning. Deficiency of Vitamin B12 often leads to silent condition of aging that appears after middle age. A Vitamin B12 deficiency develops very slowly over many years and often affects the brain and nervous system entirely. Commonly a B12 deficiency mimics 'senility', dementia or alzheimer's disease. Older people suffer several neurological symptoms including memory loss, which improves when treated with Vitamin B12. The sooner a B12 deficiency is corrected, the better it is. Delaying as much as a year may be too late to totally stop or reverse the damage caused.

One should not wait for the symptoms of Vitamin B12 deficiency to occur, since it has awful consequences and creeps up without warning. Taking supplements of B12 is a good insurance that can considerably cut risk.

Only animal foods, such as meat, fish, chicken and dairy products have Vitamin B12. Vegetarian people must take Vitamin B12 supplements. Older people must take 500 to 1000 mg of B12 per day.

### 5.1.1.4.2 Vitamin B6

Deficiency of Vitamin B6 leads to classic signs of aging, particularly failing immune system, declining mental status, failing heart health, various infectious diseases and even cancer. In fact B6 deficiency leads to reduced production of T cells, T helper cells and antibodies- all disease fighting substances of the immune system. In early stage, taking Vitamin B6 supplements repairs the damage caused.

Vitamin B6 boosts functioning of the immune system. The effective dose is 1.9 mg a day for women and 2.88 mg for men. Besides, Vitamin B6 is effective against homocysteine – the destroyer of blood vessels. It is found that folic acid affects one enzyme (discussed subsequently) that breaks down homocysteine. Without sufficient B6 in the blood, homocysteine can build up, damaging arteries and provoking heart attacks and strokes. B6 is also believed to hinder dangerous blood clotting.

Vitamin B6 also improves functioning of the brain. Adequate amount of B6 may retard age-related memory decline. Typical multivitamin pills contain 3 mg of B6, enough to correct deficiencies and boost immunity. Supplements of 10-50 mg of B6 a day may be needed to reduce homocysteine. Some of the foods rich in B6 are seafood, whole grain, nuts, soybean, banana, sweet potato and prunes. It is safest to stick to a dose of no more than 50 mg of B6 daily. Higher doses (500-1000 mg daily) may produce nervous system toxicity and can cause neurological symptoms.

### 5.1.1.4.3 Folic acid

Deficiency of folic acid, also called folate and folacin considerably enhances aging. Like Vitamin B12, folic acid can help an individual from deteriorating mental functioning. It also helps to lift one's mood, prevents and cures depression and turns off cancer. Just taking a folic acid supplement of 400-1000 micrograms a day could help to save an individual from a heart attack, cancer and psychiatric disturbances.

It has been found that elevated levels of a blood protein, homocysteine is considered a major risk factor for heart disease-even more significant than cholesterol. High blood hemocysteine triples the chances of a heart disease. The three B vitamins, particularly folic acid spur enzymes to metabolize or destroy homocysteine and thus keeps it in check. Deficiency of Vitamin B may lead to blocked arteries. A daily dose of 400 micrograms of folic acid checks the homocysteine very effectively. It is found that smokers need two times more folic acid (at least 600 micrograms daily) to achieve the same blood levels as non-smokers.

Folic acid can help block and even reverse cancer, even after premalignant cells are evident. Some studies show that lack of folic acid makes one more susceptible to lung, esophageal and breast cancer and polyps that precede colon cancer.

As one grows older, folic acid can help preserve mental faculties. Lack of folic acids in diet of young men signifies poor emotional stability, poor concentration, more introversion and lack of self-concentration. These conditions can be improved by taking adequate doses of folic acid for 6-8 weeks.

Foods such as dried beans, spinach and citrus fruits contain fairly high doses of folic acid. The requirements of the body can be met from the foods (mentioned above) for reducing homocysteine, supplements of folic acid are necessary. If one uses antibiotics for longer periods or frequently takes antacids at mealtime, one's ability to absorb folic acid drops significantly, irrespective of age.

### 5.1.2 Minerals

Some of the minerals like chromium, zinc, calcium, magnesium and selenium are very helpful in delaying aging.

#### 5.1.2.1 Chromium

As one grows older, the cells become less efficient in using insulin to process blood sugar. In fact, the cells become less sensitive or 'resistant' to insulin. In order to control blood sugar, the human body pours or dumps insulin in the blood. In case the insulin is too weak, blood sugar can rise. The combination of high level of dysfunctional insulin and sugar tend to destroy arteries by stimulating processes that build up plaque, leading ultimately to heart attacks and strokes. The overload of blood insulin and sugar can make an individual diabetic in mid or late life; this diabetes is generally irreversible.

It is found that chromium deficiency begets insulin resistance. Taking chromium supplements can help cure and prevent dreadful insulin imbalance. Basically, chromium revs up insulin action, improves insulin efficiency and improves blood cholesterol and triglycerides. Thus, taking chromium can help save an individual from the ravages of rapid aging by optimizing insulin activity. Everybody needs 200 micrograms of chromium a day. Taking chromium can help save an individual from heart disease, diabetes and possibly cancer.

Generally, the ill effects of chromium deficiency are mistaken for 'normal aging'.

The decline is slow and it takes years for the sign of chromium deficiency to show up. When chromium levels go down, after decades one's cholesterol goes up, insulin level goes up, HDL's go down and glucose levels go up. All this happens because of a diet with too little chromium and too much sugar. Both these are preventable. Chromium is believed to be an antiaging insurance policy for all of us.

Following are given some of the advantages of taking Chromium in diet or supplements:

- Chromium controls hazardous insulin by controlling the power of insulin to process sugar. Thus, with adequate chromium much less insulin circulates in the blood to attack artery walls, precipitating artherosclerosis. Its deficiency plunges an individual into adult-onset (Type II) diabetes. A timely intake of chromium supplements can help one overcome all the problems. A daily 200 micrograms of chromium picolinate improves insulin resistance within 2 weeks.
- It normalizes blood sugar. Studies have shown that if one has excessive blood sugar (which promotes diabetes and its after effects), chromium supplements can bring it down. Amazingly, if one has low blood sugar, chromium can bring it up. This results from chromium's ability to normalize insulin.

- Chromium lowers blood cholesterol. Studies show that chromium lowers bad-type LDL cholesterol and raises good type HDL cholesterol.
- It boosts immune functioning by making insulin more efficient. Insulin is known to help direct many immune functions, such as stimulating interferon and T-lymphocytes-white cells that destroy germs.
- It prevents heart disease. Studies have shown that insulin and blood sugar disorders (which are corrected by chromium) are far more important factors in heart diseases than high blood cholesterol.
- It boosts antiaging hormone, dehydroepiandrosterone (DHEA). In fact, high insulin levels (promoted by chromium deficiency) inhibit the production of DHEA by inhibiting the enzymes that convert a chemical into DHEA.

Taking chromium supplement may help in

- Lowering chromium insulin levels.
- Lowering triglycerides.
- Raising good type HDL cholesterol.
- Preventing artery clogging and heart disease.
- Lowering bad-type cholesterol.
- Normalizing blood sugar.
- Reducing risk of adult-onset diabetes.
- Preventing cancer growth.
- Boosting immune functioning.
- Increasing energy.
- Enhancing the production of DHEA.
- Extending life.

Chromium is difficult to get from vegetables and fruits. It should be taken in the form of supplements. Normally a supplement of 200 micrograms of chromium is necessary. However, in case of diabetes a dose of 400-800 micrograms daily is required. But this should be taken only on the advice of a doctor. Much of the premature aging can be prevented by chromium supplements taken before the age of 20-25 years.

### 5.1.2.2 Zinc

The proper functioning of the immune system is controlled by thymus gland (which is tucked in the neck behind the top of the breastbone of every human being) throughout life. The thymus gland (at birth it is bigger than the heart), which is big and robust in youth, shrivels up and loses its power as the age advances. It is found that at the age of 60, the thymus gland is usually a shadow of its early self, reflecting a rapid decline in immune functioning. The shrinkage of the thymus is the most spectacular sign of aging. Without an active thymus gland, the immune system's T cells do not mature enough to spot foreign invaders making an individual prone to infections. Also without the direction of the T cells, B cells also falter in their ability to make antibodies. Until recently, the slow decline of the thymus gland was considered to be in irreversible condition of advancing age. This accounts for much of the deteriorating immunity that comes from age. However, it is now established that this is not true. Studies show that the decline is stoppable and reversible and that the shrinking of the thymus gland is a myth. In fact, the thymus gland can be rejuvenated even late in life by the supplements of the mineral zinc.

You may be low in antiaging zinc if:

- You are a vegetarian, zinc is found mostly in meat,

seafood and poultry.
- You have cut back on meat.
- You eat lots of fibre, fibre blocks zinc absorption.
- You are past age 50 when your ability to absorb zinc is reduced.

Zinc supplements revive the functioning of the immune system and this results in cutting down the aging process and increases the life expectancy. In fact, it is never too late to prolong life. Zinc stimulates the production of gamma interferon, a substance essential for proper immune functioning. In fact, zinc provides protection against aging by functioning as an antioxidant and destroys the destructive free radicals. Its deficiency causes excessive free radical activity, cancer and forms of degenerative brain diseases.

A daily dose of 15-30 mg of zinc is enough to preserve immune functioning as one ages or to reverse the deficiencies and revitalizing the thymus gland and restoring youthful immune activity. It is difficult to get enough zinc in the diet especially for vegetarians and people who are cutting down on meat. Highest zinc is in seafood. Lean meat is also a rich source. Cereals, nuts and seeds are relatively high in zinc, but they also contain agents that reduce zinc absorption. Zinc supplements should be taken particularly around 40-50 years of age.

#### 5.1.2.3 Calcium

Our ancestors ate a lot of calcium but in present times we do not. Due to this, our bones may grow fragile and break. Also, as one grows older, the endocrine system weakens and the cell growth regulation may not work properly. This may lead an individual to age faster. One should know that calcium is much more than a bone savior. The cells need calcium for proper functioning. The hazards worsen with age, as one tends to absorb less calcium with passing years. A deficiency of calcium in fact, drags an individual into premature old age. Though it is better to consume calcium at a young age, it is never too late. Calcium has done wonders to people's health even in their eighties.

Calcium can fight aging by keeping the bones young and by saving people from high blood pressure even as one gets older. It can also reverse some of the high blood pressure damage. Calcium can help thwart proliferation of cancer prone cells. Numerous studies point out that calcium has anticancer activity. It also reduces the risk of colon cancer. Calcium is a weapon against bad cholesterol.

Best sources of calcium are yogurt, milk, broccoli and tofu. It is best to take calcium supplements. Even if an individual is on hypertension medication, calcium supplements can induce further drops in blood pressures. It takes a lot of calcium to stay young. Below is given the amount one needs every day

- Infants, birth to 6 months – 400 mg
- Infants, six months to 12 months – 600 mg
- Children, 1-10 years – 800 mg
- Children and young adults, 11-24 years –1200 -1500 mg
- Women, 25-50 years – 1000 mg
- Men, less than 25 years – 1000 mg
- Postmenopausal women –1000-1500 mg
- Women less than 65 – 1500 mg

***Source:*** National Institute of Health, USA, Expert panel, 1994.

It is important to know that calcium can be absorbed in the system only in presence of Vitamin D. Without enough Vitamin D, bones grow weaker and make women vulnerable to breast cancer and men to prostate and colon cancer. Good food sources of Vitamin D are Vitamin D - fortified milk, liver, fatty fish (salmon). Older people who are not exposed to sun need 200 iu of vitamin D. One should not consume excessive Vitamin D. It is quite toxic. A toxic daily dose of Vitamin D for adults could be as little as 2000 iu.

A good and smart antiaging practice is to take high calcium diet and take the entire recommended dose of calcium in supplements. Best antiaging results are achieved if calcium is taken before the age of 25. However it is never too late to take calcium supplements.

#### 5.1.2.4 Magnesium

Magnesium is a youth preserving mineral, especially for the heart. It protects cells against premature aging. Even a little shortage of magnesium appears to make a difference in how long one lives and how fast one ages. Also, as we age, we tend to eat diets lower in magnesium and also absorb less of it. Its deficiency can lead to clogged arteries, heart arrhythmias (irregular heart beats), heart attacks, high blood pressure and insulin resistance, possibly leading to diabetes.

Studies by a team of scientists at the center for research on human nutrition at France's National Institute of Agricultural Research, suggest that the main cause of fast aging induced by magnesium deficiency is increased by free radical activity in cells. In the absence of magnesium, the mitochondria, the energy factories of the cells particularly critical in heart function, are increasingly damaged. The result is that the cells become unable to create energy. In fact, damage to cell mitochondria is considered the number one underlying cause of aging by free radical experts.

Magnesium saves people from heart attacks. This is achieved by magnesium by preventing spasms of the coronary arteries and abnormal heart rhythms, a primary cause of sudden death. Also, magnesium helps deter formation of blood clots that help clog arteries and trigger heart attacks. Magnesium also inhibits release of thromboxane, a substance that makes blood platelets more sticky and apt to form clots. Magnesium also keeps blood vessels from constricting, thud warding off rise in blood pressure, strokes and heart attacks. Magnesium also regulates heartbeats and blood pressure effectively.

Magnesium has been found to prevent and even reverse diabetes. For keeping bones strong, one needs both calcium and magnesium (which work together) with Vitamin D. The ratio of calcium and magnesium is important. One should get at least half as much magnesium as calcium to get the best results. The antiaging attributes of magnesium are because it:

- Reduces vascular spasms
- Reduces angina (chest pain)
- Increases clot busting activity
- Inhibits blood platelets stickiness leading to clots
- Helps keep heartbeats normal
- Boosts good type of blood cholesterol (HDL)
- Suppresses triglyceroids
- Keeps free radicals away

One can get the daily requirement of magnesium (400-500 mg) from the foods rich in magnesium. These foods include whole grains, nuts, seeds and legumes. The amount of magnesium in one ounce of different food is given below.

| Food items | Amount of magnesium in mg |
|---|---|
| Pumpkin and squash kernels | 152 |
| Brown cereal | 135 |
| Almonds | 85 |
| Filberts | 85 |
| Cashews | 74 |
| Pine nuts | 66 |
| Peanuts | 51 |
| Walnuts | 48 |
| Oats | 42 |
| Pecans | 37 |
| Tofu | 29 |
| Soya beans | 25 |
| Lima beans | 15 |

If one does not eat magnesium rich foods, a supplement (200-300 mg daily) is necessary to retard premature aging. Magnesium supplements should not be taken if one has kidney problems or severe heart failure. If an individual has had a heart attack, it is advised to consult a physician before taking supplements.

### 5.1.2.5 Selenium

Selenium is regarded as a powerhouse of antioxidant and an essential trace mineral with diverse antiaging properties. If the selenium level goes down, the immune functioning goes awry and one is likely to fall prey to infections, cancer and heart disease. Besides, selenium is an essential building block for the creation of glutathione peroxidase, one of the body's most critical enzymes that neutralize free radicals, particularly those that attack fat molecules (turning them rancid). It is believed that the antiaging power of selenium is due to its ability to boost production of glutathione peroxidase, the free radical fighting enzyme.

Selenium is a powerful chemo preventive agent. People who have low level of selenium in blood and eat diets less in selenium tend to have cancers of breast, colon, liver, skin, lung and trachea. Selenium is believed to be particularly important in preventing lung cancer. Selenium appears to fight cancer by preventing mutations, repairing damaged cells and boosting immune functions.

Low blood levels of Selenium make one more vulnerable to heart disease. Selenium protects arteries by preventing platelet aggregation that tends to form blood clots, triggering heart attacks and strokes. Selenium also helps block oxidation of bad type LDL cholesterol, thought to be the main step in clogging of arteries. According to other studies, taking selenium can bring the failing immunity back to track. Selenium can also help keep the virus under control.

According to experts, selenium supplements might help contain the AIDS virus and prolong the survival in AIDS patient. In fact, in presence of enough selenium around in the cells, the AIDS virus does not replicate. Selenium relieves anxiety, depression and the feeling of getting tired. It improves the mental functioning in older people as increased blood flows to the brain.

Selenium is present in grains, sunflower, seeds, meat, seafood and garlic. The Brazil nuts, grown in selenium rich soil of the forests of the Amazon are the best source of Selenium. For anti-cancer protection one needs 100-200 microgram a day of selenium. In high doses, however, Selenium is toxic (hair loss, liver damage, joint inflammation).

## 5.2 Glutathione

Glutathione, a naturally occurring amino acid is considered to be the master antioxidant. Our cells produce it internally as part of the body's magnificently designed antioxidant to fend the free radical damage. Its main function in the body is to dispose off the free radicals that bring about the woes of aging. It protects each and every cell, tissue and organ in the body against free radicals. In fact, Glutathione determines the rate at which one ages and one's susceptibility to chronic diseases. A deficiency of glutathione in cells is the primary cause of aging. If one has lots of glutathione in blood and tissues, one lives longer and better. On the other hand, a deficiency dramatically declines an individuals functioning and one dies early. Glutathione regenerates immune cells and becomes immune efficient.

Glutathione helps antiaging by:

- Maintaining healthy immune functioning.
- Rejuvenating old and weak immune system.
- Helps to save an individual from cancer.
- Flushing free radicals out of rancid fat one eats.
- Keeping blood cholesterol from becoming oxidized and toxic.

- Helping to cure some forms of type II diabetes.
- Helping prevent muscular degeneration, an age related eye disease.

More of antiaging glutathione in the cells can be obtained by:

- **Eating glutathione** – foods with every meal. Most glutathione-rich foods are fresh and frozen fruits and vegetables. Cooking and heat processing destroys glutathione. The amount of glutathione per 100 grams of dry weight of fresh and cooked vegetables is given below.

| Vegetables | Fresh | Cooked |
|---|---|---|
| Carrots | 75 mg | 35 mg |
| Tomato juice | 169 mg | 27 mg |
| Spinach | 166 mg | 108 mg |

Walnuts are high in glutathione.

- Eating cruciferous vegetables like brussels, sprouts, cabbage, cauliflower and broccolli. Cruciferous vegetables also contain sulforaphane and iberin, both chemicals spur internal production of glutathione. Broccoli has high concentrations of preformed glutathione.
- Taking Vitamin C (500 mg per day) is a quick and easy way to be sure that cells maintain high levels of glutathione.
- Taking glutamine supplement boosts the blood levels of glutathione much better than taking glutathione directly.

- Taking Selenium supplements and high foods in selenium also stimulate increased bodily production of glutathione.
- Taking glutathione supplements with a meal is an insurance against problems of aging.

### 5.3 Coenzyme Q-10

Coenzyme Q-10 also known as ubiquinol–10 or Vitamin Q is one of the brightest new antioxidants which help in postponing aging and preventing or treating age-related diseases, namely heart diseases. It is a natural substance produced by the body and is also found in certain foods like seafood. It helps defeat the ravages of aging and prolonging life. For anyone over 50 years of age, taking coenzyme Q-10 supplements could reenergize aging tissues, alleviating the effects of aging process and age associated disease.

Coenzyme Q-10 is an antioxidant similar to Vitamin E and protects fat molecules from becoming oxidized or infused with free radicals. Co Q-10 is vital in keeping all cells intact, functional and alive. Co Q-10 is highly concentrated in heart muscle cells, which need tremendous amount of energy to keep a healthy heart pumping some one thousand times a day.

Coenzyme Q-10 helps to fight aging. It

- Saves arteries by striking at the root cause of artherosclerosis. It is very strong in halting the oxidation of blood cholesterol, which is the first step in making a rotten mess in arteries, precipitating heart attacks and strokes. It destroys LDL bad type cholesterol better than Vitamin E or even better than beta carotene.

- Revives failing hearts. During congestive heart failure, the heart muscles become weak and the heart is enlarged and is too weak to pump enough blood. This is all due to deficiency of Co Q-10. Supplements of Co Q-10 revives the failing hearts also in elderly patients.
- Lowers blood pressure. Co Q-10 help lower blood pressure by taking about 225 mg daily.
- Boosts immune functioning.
- Protects brain from damage.

Coenzyme Q-10 is used as anti-factor and for the protection of heart in a number of countries like USA, Israel, Italy, Sweden and Japan.

Co Q-10 should always be taken with a little fat such as peanut butter or olive oil for better absorption. The best sources of Co Q-10 are fatty fish (like mackerel and sardines), organ meats (such as heart, liver and kidney) soy oil and peanuts. The production of Co Q-10 in the body is enhanced by taking Vitamin E, selenium and B vitamins (B6, B12, B2, niacin and folic acid)

## 5.4 Herbal Therapy

A herbal extract (or concentrate pressed into tablets) is commonly used in USA and other parts of the world (particularly Germany) to treat any kind of circulating problems including mental faculties that come with age. The antiaging agent is present in the extract of leaves of ginkgo tree (called ginkgo biloba), an ornamental tree that grows in temperate climate throughout the world including USA. Its leaf, pulverised into a powder or liquid (or pressed into tablets) has been used for a long time due to its antiaging effects on the brain. It takes about 50 pounds of dried leaves to make one pound of ginkgo biloba extract that is used as a liquid or capsule or is pressed into tablets.

The antiaging property of Ginkgo is due to its ability to improve blood circulation. This is very important to elderly whose blood vessels are typically not old, inflexible and clogged.

In fact, ginkgo encourages blood to squeeze through even the tiniest, narrowed vessels to nourish oxygen-starved tissue in the brain, heart and limbs. It also restores memory and wipes away muscle pain. A number of scientific findings confirm that ginkgo stimulates blood flow feeding oxygen to tissues, most likely by dilating blood vessels and discouraging blood platelets from sticking together and forming clots. In fact, ginkgo delivers blood even to disease-damaged areas, bringing new life to an aging brain.

Ginkgo is a potent antioxidant, even stronger than Vitamin E in scavenging free radicals, thus blocking highly destructive oxidation of fatty cell membranes. In Europe, ginkgo is being used for improving the quality of life for the elders. The antiaging effect of ginkgo (on the basis of a number of studies) is attributed to

- Improved blood flow through arteries, veins and capillaries.
- Improved failing memory in the elderly.
- Slowing the progression of alzheimers disease.
- Reducing leg pain from diminishing blood flow to limbs.
- Inhibiting bacterial activity involved in gum disease.
- Reviving dizziness or vertigo.

- Reducing ringing in the ears (tinnitus).
- Inhibiting deteriorating vision due to oxygen deprivation of the retina.
- Improving hearing loss related to reduced blood flow.
- Lowering blood pressure.
- Raising good type HDL cholesterol.
- Inhibiting abnormal blood clotting.

Ginkgo is available in most of the countries in tablet form. It contains certain compounds called – flavone glycosides to the extent of 24-25%. The usual dose is 40-mg ginkgo tablet thrice daily to relieve aging problems.

## 5.5 Garlic

Garlic, a natural ancient wonder drug is known for about 5000 years as a health tonic and a curing agent for a large number of ailments. If one wants to live longer and more vital, the body cells should be fed with garlic. The bulb of garlic is packed with about 400 chemicals including many antioxidants, which give it a potent activity to guard cells from damage and the entire body from premature aging. It is not clear as to which substance in garlic has the most profound effects. However it is for sure that the chemicals present in garlic have a range of talents–as antibiotics, antiviral agents, cholesterol reducers, anticoagulants, blood pressure reducers, cancer inhibitors, anti-inflammatory agents and also protectors of aging brain cells. Some of the beneficial effects of garlic are:

- It blocks and strife cancer. People who eat garlic are less apt to get certain cancers such as stomach and colon. Garlic may not just save people from getting cancer but prolong their life after they have it. It inhibits cancer in all tissues.

- Its antioxidant powers block free radicals from oxidizing bad type LDL cholesterol, thus crippling its ability to clog arteries.
- It also lowers blood pressure. Taking two garlic cloves a day for 2–3 months, reduces the blood pressure from 170/102 to 150/90.
- It fights clot by discouraging formation of dangerous clots or 'thinning the blood'. In fact, garlic prevents platelets from sticking to each other or the walls of arteries, a first step in the clotting of arteries. Besides, garlic also revs up the clot dissolving fibrolytic system. Cooked garlic seems to have even more antithrombotic activity.
- It prevents heart attacks. Even after one has had a heart attack or a heart disease, eating garlic may help to save an individual. In fact, garlic helps to dissolve blockages in arteries, partially damaged by atherosclerosis.
- Rejuvenates brain and immunity. The two faculties that are brain and immune system which are known to deteriorate with age can be rejuvenated. It is also effective in Alzheimer's like "sensility'. The Ukrainian remedy for old age debility is to take one spoonful at night of a preparation made by grinding one pound of garlic and mixing it with juice of about 24 lemons and leaving it covered for 24 days.
- Delays aging.
- Garlic extract has been found to have 'beta blocker' activity (beta blockers are well known heart and

blood pressure drugs) by decreasing the strength and frequency of vascular muscle contraction.

- Garlic has anti-stress, anti-anxiety antidepressant activities. It is believed that garlic affects the release of serotonin, a ubiquitous brain chemical involved in resulting moods and behaviour, including anxiety, depression, pain, aggression, stress, sleep and memory. In fact, higher levels of serotonin in the brain tend to act as a tranquilizer to calm down people.

Garlic can be taken in raw form (if one can tolerate its odor and smell) or cooked form. Even garlic powder is good enough. However, cooking and crushing change garlic's power. The well-known garlic pills available everywhere are as good as fresh garlic. One may consume 1-3 cloves a day for anti-aging effects. In supplements, 600-800 mg of garlic powder per day has heart protective effects. About 1-2 cloves of garlic blocked the formation of carcinogenic nitro amines in the stomach. The antiaging potency of garlic depends on the size of the clove and the soil in which it is grown. Garlic grown in selenium rich soil is particularly rich in selenium, which enhances the antiaging powers. Alternatively, a combination of garlic and selenium supplement does the same job.

To sum up, the anti-aging properties of garlic is attributed to its ability to:

- Reviving immune system.
- Reducing high blood cholesterol.
- Anticoagulant action to thin the blood and discourage dangerous blood clots.
- Protecting aging brains from mental malfunction

including memory loss, diminished thinking, depression and dementia.

- Inhibiting cell chances leading to cancer and also help to destroy cancer cells.
- Checking free radical damage in cells.

## 5.6 Fruits and Vegetables

These are considered as a miracle diet for antiaging. The key to slow aging is to increase the ability of cells to resist destruction from free radicals. The best course is to destroy or neutralize the free radicals as soon as they are formed. This can be achieved basically by antioxidants. There is only one place where one finds various types of antioxidants. This is in fruits and vegetables. The fruits and vegetables have magnificent powers to transform the lives of cells and destiny, at all times and specially at the time of growing old. It is not possible to pin point one or two antioxidants (chemical substances) present in fruits and vegetables, which are responsible for combating the avages of aging. Many experts believe (and correctly so) that many constituents in fruits and vegetables collaborate to combat the ravages of aging. The only sure and best way to get the total anti-aging advantage is to eat fruits and vegetables in their whole, complex or original form. Fruits and vegetables prevent premature aging by:

- Blocking cancer. The antioxidant present in vegetables like cabbage, broccoli, cauliflower and other cruciferous vegetables neutralize the free radicals, which in a way are responsible for cancer. Also, the chemicals present in the above vegetables speed the removal of harmful estrogen from the body, thwarting breast cancer. It is found that tomato eaters are five times less likely to develop pancreatic cancer. In fact, even after the cancer is diagnosed, eating lots of vegetables and fruits can hinder the progress of cancer. It is in fact, never too late to lower the risk of a future cardiovascular event or even cancer by eating more fruits and vegetables.

- Preventing cardiovascular disease. A number of studies have shown that eating lots of fruits and vegetables can save us from not only heart attack, but also even help clear or 'unclog' the arteries after heart attacks and strokes. A rich diet in fruits and vegetables also help lower high blood pressure. It is on record that a number of high blood pressure patients after eating lots of fruits and vegetables for 2-3 months regularly did not need drugs to lower their high blood pressure.
- Preserving mental and physical faculties. Some studies suggest that lycopene, an antioxidant present in tomatoes preserve mental and physical faculties. So one should take lot of tomatoes. Lycopene is also present in watermelon and to a slight extent in apricots. Also, a lack of folic acid, concentrated in green leafy vegetables as well as legumes is also associated with failing mental faculties and depression.
- Vitamin C and folic acid rich in fruits and vegetables seem to combat free radical damage that cause the opacity of the lens known as cataract. Spinach is also likely to save an individual from another vision destroying disease of aging, macular degeneration that results from years of

free radical damage to retina.

One can indeed slow down aging by the following:

- Eat 5-10 servings of fruits and vegetables daily. One serving is one half cup cooked or chopped raw fruit or vegetables. Take one cup of raw leafy vegetables, one medium piece of fruit or six ounces of fruit or vegetable juice.
- Eat lots of different fruits and vegetables, since it is the combination of antioxidants (chemical substances) that give the most powerful protection.
- Chose fresh and frozen fruits and vegetables over canned ones whenever possible.
- Eat whole fruits, vegetables and juices. Juice, extracted from fruits and vegetables contains antiaging substances but not the entire spectrum found in whole fruit or vegetable. The best is to blend the entire fruit or vegetable using a high-powered blender so as to obtain fine pulp, which will give much more protection than the juice.
- As far as possible chose deep colored fruits and vegetables. More and better antioxidants are present in such fruits and vegetables. For example, the darkest orange, carrots and sweet potatoes and deepest green leafy vegetables such as spinach and lettuce contain the most antioxidant caroteniods, including beta-carotene and lutein. Red grapes, red onions and yellow onions have much more antioxidant quercetin than green grapes and white onions. Blueberries contain high concentration of antioxidant flavonoids.
- As far as possible vegetables should be lightly cooked to retain most of the antioxidants,

steaming, grilling and stir-frying vegetables generally preserve more antioxidants than by heavy boiling. Microwaving destroys about 15-20% of antioxidants.

Practically all fruits and vegetables contribute to delaying aging (the only precaution is that as far as possible one should take whole fruits and vegetables in raw form. However, vegetables if cooked should be lightly cooked).

Following are given some of the vegetables and fruits (called super antiaging vegetables and fruits) which are very good insurance against aging. One should not ignore them.

***Cabbage:***

It is a cruciferous vegetable with potent antioxidant activity. It prevents cancers of colon, stomach and breast. An antioxidant in cabbage, indole-3-carbinol, accelerates the disposal of a harmful form of estrogen that promotes breast cancer. For best advantage one should eat cabbage raw or lightly cooked.

***Broccoli:***

It contains a number of antioxidants. An antioxidant called sulforaphane present in broccoli revved up the activity of detoxification enzymes that slashed cancer rates by about 66%. Broccoli is packed with free radicals destroyers' Vitamin C, beta-carotene, quercetin, glutathione and lutein. It is also a rich source of trace metal chromium, a life extender and protector against the ravages of out of control insulin and blood sugar. Eating broccoli has even been linked to longer survival in lung cancer patients.

*Carrots:*

Carrots are the best in preventing aging. A large number of studies suggest that the yellow pigment, beta-carotene present in carrots is one of the best antioxidant. Beta-carotene cuts lung cancer risks in half, even among former heavy smokers. Beta-carotene also boosts immune functioning. Carrot juice is the best. One cup contains 24 mg of beta-carotene.

*Onions:*

Onions are a kind of garlic (a super antiaging food that can also be taken in a pill form) and have a number of antiaging activity. These are full of antioxidants and help prevent cancer, especially stomach cancer, 'thin the blood', discourage clots and raise good type HDL cholesterol. Red and yellow onions (not white onions) are the richest source of quercetin, a well-known antioxidant that inactivates cancer-causing agents, inhibits enzymes that spur cancer growth, has anti-inflammatory, antibacterial, anti-fungal and antiviral activity. Quercetin also keeps bad LDL cholesterol from turning toxic and attacking arteries.

*Spinach:*

The leafy vegetable, spinach is packed with a variety of antioxidants and is helpful in warding off a broad variety of free radical inspired diseases including cancer, heart disease, high blood pressure, strokes, cataracts and even psychiatric problems. Lutein, an antioxidant present in spinach is as good as beta-carotene. Spinach is rich in both lutein and beta-carotene. It is also rich in folic acid, a brain and artery protector, as well serves as an anticancer agent.

*Tomatoes:*

These are the richest and the only reliable source of a remarkable antioxidant, lyopene, which is more powerful in snuffing out specific free radicals than even beta-carotene. In the elderly, lycopene preserves mental and physical functioning. It also reduces the risk of pancreatic and cervical cancers. Two other tomato chemicals—p-cumaric acid and chlorogenic acid—suppress formation of cancer causing nitrosamines. Cooking tomatoes does not destroy lycopene.

*Avacado:*

It is abundant in glutathione, the master antioxidant, which among other miracles, help neutralize highly destructive fat in food. Though avacado is high in fat, most of it is a good fat - monounsaturated, a type that resists oxidation. Eating avacados also lowers and improves blood cholesterol. It is also rich in potassium, which protects blood vessels.

*Berries:*

Most of the berries (blue berries, cranberries, strawberries, and raspberries) are loaded with antioxidants, which save cells from premature aging. Blue berries, have more antioxidants called anthocyanin's than any other food. Both blue berries and cranberries help ward off urinary tract infections. Blue berries lower the rate of all kinds of cancer. Berries are particularly rich in the antioxidant Vitamin C.

*Citrus fruits:*

The well known citrus fruit, orange is full of antioxidants and is called a natural anticancer inhibitor known. The antioxidants present are Vitamin C flavanoids, carotenoids and terpenes. Grape fruit also has a unique type of fibre (especially in the membranes and juice sacs) that dramatically reduces cholesterol and even reverse the aging disease artherosclerosis. Grape fruit is also a rich source of glutathione (the master antioxidant) that fights all kinds of free radical damage to cells and thus prevents aging.

*Grapes:*

Grapes contain about twenty known antioxidants that work together to fend off oxygen free radicals attacks that promote disease and aging. The antioxidants in grapes are present in the skin and seeds. The more colorful the skin, the greater the antioxidant content. This implies that red and purple grapes are more powerful. The antioxidants in grapes have anti clogging activity, inhibit oxidation of LDL cholesterol and relax blood vessels. The antioxidant quercetin (also plentiful in onions) is the foremost antiaging component.

Resins, which are simply dried grapes, contain higher concentrations of anticlogging compounds than fresh grapes.

### 5.6.1 Vegetarians live longer

It is definite that eating more fruits and vegetables and less meat (or cutting down on meat) can overcome the consequences of aging and prolong life. The life can be stretched to a maximum by eating only plant foods (vegetables and fruits) and seafood. In general, vegetarians weigh less, have lower cholesterol and blood pressure and experience fewer heart attacks and cancers and have stronger immune systems.

## 5.7 Eat Fish

There is absolutely no doubt that fish eaters are more apt to escape aging diseases, such as heart disease, cancer, arthritis, diabetes, psoriasis and bronchitis. Also, fish eaters around the world live longer. The Japanese who hold the world's record for longevity, eat maximum amount of fish. The reason is that all sea food but fatty fish in particular, such as salmon, tuna, mackerel and sardines are rich in a peculiar type of fat called omega - 3, fatty acids, which protects arteries by 'thinning the blood' (like aspirin), thus discoursing blood clotting that triggers heart attack and strokes. Such marine fat also lowers blood pressure and triglycerides, a potentially dangerous blood fat, raises good type HDL cholesterol, regulates heartbeats, makes aged arteries more flexible and helps block inflammatory process that promote arthritis, cancer, psoriasis, diabetes and general cell dysfunctions. Besides, seafood is also rich in powerful antioxidants, including selenium and ubiqunol (coenzyme Q-10) that fight diseases and general aging. Salmon, mackerel and sardines are especially high in coenzyme Q-10.

You can add years to life and defy death by taking up fish eating, even if one already has a heart disease. Fish oil keeps arteries young (less clogged). Fish oil is one of the world's most reliable ways of slashing triglycerides, a dangerous blood fat. In fact taking fish oil or eating salmon raises good type HDL cholesterol. Eating a mere one-ounce of fish a day cuts one's chances of having a heart attack to half. Taking 3000 mg of fish oil a day (the amount in seven ounces of mackerel) make stiffened, aged arteries significantly more flexible, allowing them to stretch better in response to changes in blood pressure. Fish eating also curtails strokes and wards off diabetes Type II. It thwarts colon cancer and blocks breast cancer and also protect smoker's lungs.

One can get the antiaging fish oil by eating fish with the most antiaging omega—3 fatty acids like mackerel, salmon and tuna. Particularly avoid eating omega—6 fatty acids as in corn oil and regular sunflower oil. These are most apt to neutralize fish powers in cells by spewing off lots of free radicals that can damage cells. If one eats fish every day, one should be sure to take Vitamin E capsules (200-400 iu daily) to preserve optimum immune functioning.

One can also get life saving omega—3 fatty acids in certain plant foods. Exceptionally high in Omega—3 fatty acids are wheat germ oil, canola oil, walnut, soybeans and flaxseed oil. The plant omega—3 fatty acids are the only alternatives for vegetarians, but they are less biologically active than omega-3 fatty acids in fish oil. Following are given the plants, which contain omega—3 fatty acids.

| High | Grams of omega—3 fatty acid per 100 grams |
|---|---|
| Wheat germ oil | 6.9 |
| Butternuts | 8.7 |
| Walnut oil | 10.4 |
| Canola oil | 11.1 |
| Flaxseed oil | 53.3 |

| Medium | Grams of omega-3 fatty acid per 100 grams |
|---|---|
| Oat germ | 1.4 |
| Beech nuts | 1.7 |
| Soybeans, kernels, roasted | 1.5 |
| Soybeans, green | 3.2 |
| Soybean oil | 6.8 |
| Walnuts | 6.8 |

Source: US Department of Agriculture.

### 5.8 Soybeans

Soybean is an antiaging pill having powerful antioxidants that can perform magic in cells. It slows the pace with which one ages. Soybeans interfere with free radical damage on which depends how fast one ages. This explains why Japanese who eat the maximum soybeans in the world live longer than anyone.

Soybean is infact a powerhouse of antioxidants and other agents including genistein, diadzein, protease inhibitors, saponins, phytosterols, phenolic acids and lecithins most of which battle against the chronic diseases. For example, a protease inhibitor in soybeans, called Bowman-Birk inhibitor is versatile against various cancers. Also the amino acids in soybeans are less vulnerable to oxidation, so unlike many other foods, soybeans don't spew scads of damaging free radicals throughout one's body to mangle and age one's cells.

Soybeans are a rare source of high concentration of a wonder drug, called genistein, which is a potent/ antioxidant with wide ranging biological antiaging and anticancer activities. It curbs the growth of all types of cancer cells–of the breast, colon, lung, prostate, skin and blood (leukemia).

Genistein saves arteries since it obstructs proliferation of smooth muscle cells in artery walls that promotes plaque built up and clogged arteries. It also clamps down on the activity of the enzyme, thrombin that promotes blood clotting leading to heart attacks and strokes. Another soybean compound, diadzein has some but not all the genistein's powers. Diadzen, like genistein is also an isoflavone and blocks cancer in animals.

Soybeans prevents breast cancer, blocks prostate cancer, saves arteries, regulates blood sugar, builds strong bones and in this way is helpful for prolongation of life and prevent aging. To get antiaging benefits of soybeans, eat the beans proteins as found in soymilk, soy flour, the whole beans, and tofu. In fact, to keep the cells constantly supplied with soy chemicals, genistein and daidzein, one should eat soybean foods daily. The antiaging soy can be taken in the following terms:

- For making chapattis, use a mixture of soy flour and wheat flour in the ratio 1:2
- Use soymilk (defatted) in your cereal
- Use roasted soy nuts as a snack
- Use tofu in place of cheese
- Cook green soybeans as a vegetable
- Take soybeans soup

## 5.9 Tea

It is commonly known as the longevity drink. Tea is an extraordinary drink—because it is made from the leaves of *camellia sinesis,* a warm weather evergreen plant, containing a number of antioxidants that are dissolved into hot water when one makes tea. Number of different types of tea, viz., black, green, oolong—all boost your chances of reaching old age in good shape according to new research. Drinking antioxidant packed tea delays aging, prolonging life and scaring off many chronic diseases including cancer and heart disease. A number of studies identified tea drinking as an insurance against disease and premature death.

Tea can be considered as a chemical soup of a number of antioxidant polyphenols such as catechins and quercetin (also concentrated in grapes, berries and onions). A number of studies indicate that drinking tea peps up antioxidant activity in one's blood. Tea also neutralizes cell destroying nitrosamines derived from cured meats and hetrocyclic amines formed when meat is cooked. This implies that drinking tea at the same time as eating meat may defuse some of the dangers.

To get the maximum antioxidant activity, tealeaves should be allowed to stay in hot water for about 3 minutes. All caffeine is released in the first minute of brewing. Tea is believed (on the basis of number of studies) to prevent cardiovascular deaths, stifles cancer and keeps gum healthy.

# 6

# Beware of the Stuff that Robs You of Your Health

We have now seen that in our system there is a continuous fight going on between the free radicals and antioxidants (the neutralizers of the free radicals). In case the free radicals win, we lead a path of aging. However, if the antioxidants have their way, we are sure to live a healthy, disease free, happy and long life. In view of this it is extremely important to choose the right type of foods and beverages. Following are given some of the guidelines which one should follow for delaying the aging process.

## 6.1 Fats

We know that eating fat makes one not only gain weight but also ruin one's arteries leading to heart attack, stroke and a number of other conditions (ailments) including cancer. The alarming crime of fat is less well known. It makes one age much faster and makes one look old. Thus, the speed by which one ages (fast or slow aging) depends on the type of fat one eats.

Fat, an important component of our daily nutrition provides more than twice the energy compared to a gram of carbohydrate or protein. (a gram of fat provides 9 calories compared to a gram of carbohydrate or protein which provides 4 calories.) Fat is required in the body to manufacture hormones, build cell membranes and also for movement of vitamins throughout the body. The accumulated fat is a source of energy for the body. However, the amount of fat consumed, directly affects the body's cholesterol level, since the fat interacts with liver to make cholesterol. A high fat diet can raise cholesterol levels and lead to coronary heart disease, the number one killer. High fat diet may also increase the risk of many cancers, including those of colon, breast, prostate, ovary, uterus and skin. In fact, only a small amount of fat is required to keep a balance in the body.

The fats in general are of three types. These are:

*(i)* **Saturated fats:** found in meat, fish, poultry, eggs, nuts, whole fat dairy products, palm and coconut oil. The saturated fats are usually solid at room temperature. On the basis of various studies, it has been shown that a variety of cancers including colon, prostrate, lung and breasts are associated with the high intake of saturated fats.

*(ii)* **Polyunsaturated fats:** are found in corn oil, cottonseed oil, sesame oil, sunflower oil and soybeans. These are usually liquid at room temperature and are not as risky as saturated fats but should be kept to a minimum.

*(iii)* **Monounsaturated fats:** are found in olive oil, canola oil and peanut oil. These are also present in avocados, olives and nuts like almonds, peanuts, cashews and pecone. These do not cause an increase in blood cholesterol levels as other fats do. It is found that certain sections of populations,

particularly in Italy, Greece, Spain and southern parts of India use monounsaturated fats and have a low incidence of cancer and cardiovascular disease. The polysaturated fats are better than saturated fats and monounsaturated fats are better than polyunsaturated fats. In view of this it is best to use monounsaturated fats like olive oil or peanut oil.

There are several theories as to the mechanism by which fats might instigate or assist in the growth of tumors.

- By using fats, the body produce free radicals, which can damage the DNA
- Secretion of bile acids into the intestines increases and this may be converted into carcinogenic compounds in the colon (Bile acids produced by the liver normally help the body to digest fats)
- Fats interfere with the body's signals to cells, to stop dividing
- Making cells less susceptible to defend against invaders.

Those who eat red meat daily are more than 2 to 3 times likely to get cancer than those who eat red meat less than once a month. Eating vegetable fat or fat from dairy foods does not increase the risk. Experts believe that not more than about 30% of the total daily calories should come from saturated fats like butter. The calculations become easier if 30% of calories from fat are 53 grams of fat in a 1,600 calories diet. However, if a person is suffering from any type of cancer or any cardiovascular disease, it is necessary that the total dietary fat intake be not more than 10% of the calories and also to avoid all types of food that contain cholesterol.

One should follow the following guidelines for the consumption of fats:

**1. Cut down on meat consumption**

- Cut down the meat, poultry and other animal products.
- Eat a meatless or low meat diet several times a week.
- Select skinless white meat chicken or turkey rather than dark.
- Select good grades of meat which contain less fat.
- Trim away all visible fat from meat and remove skin and visible fat before cooking.

The most important reason for reducing amount of meat is that it is one of the greatest sources of dioxan, a toxic chemical that may be responsible for a large number of cases of cancer. Dioxan, produced by incinerators, chemical processing, chlorine bleaching of paper and pulp and the burning diesel fuel, unusually gets released into the atmosphere. The particles settle on crops and vegetation and are consumed by livestock and poultry.

**2. Select foods that are low in fat**

- These include fruits, vegetables and most grains, breads and starches such as rice, potatoes and pasta.
- Select reduced fat meals.
- Buy fish either fresh or packed in water, not in oil.

**3. Use low fat and not fat dairy products**

- Use skimmed milk or 1% fat milk rather than whole milk. Use low fat or non-fat cheese and yogurt.
- Cut down on salad dressings.
- Opt for tomato or vegetable based preparations rather than cream based recipes.

- Use butter or margarine sparingly.

**4. Use low fat cooking methods**

- Broiling, baking, steaming, micro waving, roasting and stir-frying all help to avoid fatty cooking oils.
- Use non-stick cookware so as to reduce considerably the use of oil.
- Eat fried foods sparingly.

**One should know that**

- Fats major crime against humanity is not heart disease or obesity, but accelerated aging.
- The worst fats are polyunsaturated fats and cholesterol.
- The monounsaturated fats such as olive oil are the best and are called longevity fats.
- The most dangerous fats are in corn oil and sunflower oil.

Following are given some of the edible oils ranked from worst to best by the percentage of omega-6 polysaturated fatty acids.

| Oil | % | |
|---|---|---|
| Safflower oil | 77% | Bad (Polysaturated) |
| Sunflower oil | 69% | |
| Corn oil | 61% | |
| Soybean oil | 54% | |
| Walnut oil | 51% | Quality of the edible oil |
| Sesame seed oil | 41% | |
| Peanut oil | 33% | |
| Canola oil | 22% | |
| Flaxseed oil | 16% | |
| Olive oil | 8% | |
| Macadamia nut oil | 3% | Good (monosaturated) |

Some safflower and sunflower seed oils have been altered to make them highly monosaturated instead of polysaturated. So check the label before use.

Following are given some of the fats that make one age faster (become old) and make one age slower (look young)

| Fats that make one older and age faster | Fats that make one age slowly or keeps one young |
|---|---|
| Highly unsaturated fats such as corn, safflower, sunflower, sunflower seed, peanut oils. | Olive oil<br>Canola oil |
| Margarine or shortening (trans fatty acids) | Macadamia nut oil |
| Animal fats in meat, poultry, dairy products | Fish oil<br>Flaxseed oil |

The best antioxidant fat is olive oil (and other monosaturated fats) to make the aging process slower. Avoid hydrogenated soybean oils; use plain soybean oil sparingly. However, soy proteins are good.

### 6.2 Avoid Taking Meat

Making meat the main dish in every meal is a good way to grow old fast. Substitute main dishes by vegetables, grain, legumes and pasta. Eating meat sabotages one's cells, promoting aging along with heart damage and cancer. In case one likes to eat meat following guidelines for its consumption should be observed.

- Eat a low meat meal 2-3 times a week.
- Select skinless white meat chicken or turkey rather than red meat.
- Select good grades of meat, which contain less fat.
- Trim away all visible fat from meat and remove skin and visible fat before cooking.
- The most important reason for reducing the amount of meat is that it is one of the greatest source of dioxan, a toxic chemical that causes a variety of cancers, including colon, prostrate, lung and breast. These are associated with the high intake of fat.
- The antiaging effects of meat can be overcome to a certain extent with antioxidants by cooking with garlic.
- Eat good quality fish.

However, the best way for prolonging life and slowing aging is not to take meat.

### 6.3 Excessive Alcoholic Drinks

Alcohol is most widely used in practically all societies. It can be procured from the local market. In fact, alcohol is responsible for about 3% of all cancer deaths; this is attributed to excessive use of alcohol. Consuming excessive alcoholic drinks is a sure way to reduce one's life span and growing old fast. Some other harmful effects of alcohol are:

*(i)* It activates chemical carcinogens

*(ii)* It causes nutritional deficiencies

*(iii)* It decreases body's capacity to fight diseases including cancer, Aids and heart ailments.

*(iv)* It suppresses the immune system

*(v)* It irritates organ lining.

A common belief amongst people who consume alcohol is that 'hard' liquor is more harmful than beer or wine (whiskey has an alcohol content of 40-50% or 90-100 'proof ' as compared to 3-6% in beer). Because alcoholic beverages contain other chemical compounds, proof alcohol does not determine co-carcinogenicity. How much one drinks is more important than what one drinks. On the basis of studies (1990 report) carried out on a large number of Japanese, it was found that increased risk of rectal cancer was associated with wine and beer consumption but not with consumption of hard liquor. In a similar study (1981) in USA it was found that those who consumed hard liquor had higher rates of esophageal cancer than those who consumed an equivalent amount of wine or beer.

One thing is clear that alcohol and tobacco together greatly compound the risk of all cancers. The best solution is to avoid drinking alcohol. This can be easily done by ordering for mineral water, club soda, fruit juice, vegetable juice etc. whenever put in the company of alcohol consumers. However, if one is forced to take an alcoholic beverage, keep the following tips (as suggested by the American Institute for Cancer Research, USA) in mind:

- Eat before you drink and while you drink. Alcohol enters the blood stream faster when the stomach is empty, enhancing its effects
- Take diluted drinks
- One should never take alcohol when feeling

thirsty. Quench your thirst with water or juice then sip alcoholic beverages slowly.

People who consume more than two alcoholic beverages a day are classified as alcohol abusers. The American Medical Association, USA has recognized (1956) alcoholism as a disease.

It is best for an alcoholic person to consult a physician or specialist for alcohol—abuse treatment. The question is—how to assess an alcoholic? If any of the following signs are seen in an individual she/he may be called an alcoholic:

- Greater amount of alcohol consumed at frequent intervals.
- Feeling uncomfortable when alcohol is not available.
- Making excuses to family and friends for drinking.
- Start drinking early in the day.
- Experiencing a blackout (episodes of total memory loss).
- Experiencing hallucinations or phobias.
- Consuming alcohol for days together.

Alcoholics, in their own interest should consult a qualified physician or alcohol—abuse counselor who can help them determine the appropriate therapy.

## 6.4 Excessive Calories Intake

Excessive intake of calories makes you obese. Besides, it increases considerably risk of heart diseases, cancer, diabetes etc. Controlling the intake of calories help prolong life and also slow down considerably the aging process. Following is given some advice on how to restrict calories to prolong life:

- Cut back calories gradually so that you lose body weight very slowly.
- The sooner you start a calorie-restricted diet after you are fully grown, the better.
- Have the most nutrients from fruits and vegetables.

It is well known that keeping healthy reduces the risk of cancer, cardiovascular diseases and other ailments. The way to keep healthy is to take nutritious food and keep the intake of calories as per the requirement of body. The body weight also depends in part on the calories one takes. Of course, a very active person, for example, a competitive athlete can burn a large number of calories without gaining weight. But for most people a high-calorie diet adds extra body fat. Being overweight increases the risks of cancers of breast, kidney, cole rectum, gallbladder, cervix, uterus, ovaries and prostrate. Excess body fat increases ovarian cancer because it metabolizes the hormone estrogen, which stimulates cell growth in these organs. A number of theories have been postulated on how body fat and high calorie diet affect some cancers. One is that chemical carcinogens are stored in body fat rather than being expelled from the body. Another theory is that the energy supply from calories exerts some control over the rate of cell multiplication.

The most important question that arises is, how many calories are needed each day to maintain one healthy and within normal weight individual. The number of calories needed per day depends on one's height, body frame and activity level.

Proceed as follows:

*(i)* Measure your height (without shoes)

*(ii)* Find your body frame. This can be determined by any of the following two methods:

(a) Place your thumb and the index fingers of one hand around your other wrist (smallest part closest to your hand). You have a

- **Small frame:** if thumb and index finger overlap
- **Medium frame:** if thumb and index finger just touch
- **Large frame:** if thumb and index finger do not meet

(b) Measure your wrist at the smallest area, nearest to your hand. Find out your body frame by your wrist measurement, and your height by referring to the following Table 6.1.

**Table 6.1. Body frame based on wrist measurement**

| | | Wrist measurement | |
|---|---|---|---|
| **Height** | **Small Frame** | **Medium Frame** | **Large Frame** |
| <5' 3" | <5' ½" | 5' ½"-5' ¾" | >5' ¾" |
| 5' 3"-5' 4" | <6' ½" | 6"-6' ¾" | >6' ¼" |
| >5' 4" | <6' ¼" | 6' ¼"-6' ½" | >6' ½" |

***Note:*** You can convert height in inches to height in centimeter by multiplying by 2.54.

*(iii)* Activity level

The activity level depends on the activities one performs. One can find their activity level by the Table 6.2.

**Table. 6.2. Activity level**

| Level of activity | Type of activity engaged in |
|---|---|
| Very little activity | Sitting, standing like working in a laboratory, driving, typing, sewing, ironing, cooking, playing cards, playing a musical instrument. |
| Light activity | Walking (2.5-3 mph), house cleaning, child care, golf, sailing, table tennis. |
| Moderate activity | Walking (3.5-4 mph), carrying a load, cycling, skiing, tennis, dancing. |
| Heavy activity | Walking uphill with a load, heavy manual labour such as digging, climbing, basketball, football, soccer. |

Finally using your height, body frame and level of activity find out the approximate number of calories you need to maintain desirable weight by referring to tables given for men (Table 6.3) and women (Table 6.4).

**Table 6.3. Desireable weights and calorie levels for men**

| Height without Shoes | Frame Size | Desirable Weight (pound) | Calorie Level Based on Physical Activity | | | |
|---|---|---|---|---|---|---|
| | | | Very Light(Calorie) | Light(Calorie) | Moderate(Calorie) | Heavy(Calorie) |
| 5'5" | Small | 129 (124- 133) | 1,700 | 1,950 | 2,200 | 2,600 |
| | Medium | 137 (130 -143) | 1,800 | 2,050 | 2,350 | 2,750 |
| | Large | 147 (138- 156) | 1,900 | 2,200 | 2,500 | 2,950 |
| 5'6" | Small | 133 (128- 137) | 1,750 | 2,000 | 2,250 | 2,650 |
| | Medium | 141 (134 -147) | 1,850 | 2,100 | 2,400 | 2,800 |
| | Large | 152 (142- 161) | 2,000 | 2,300 | 2,600 | 3,050 |
| 5'7" | Small | 137 (132- 141) | 1,800 | 2,050 | 2,350 | 2,750 |
| | Medium | 145 (138 -152) | 1,900 | 2,200 | 2,450 | 2,900 |
| | Large | 157 (147- 166) | 2,050 | 2,350 | 2,650 | 3,150 |
| 5'8" | Small | 141 (136- 145) | 1,850 | 2,100 | 2,400 | 2,850 |
| | Medium | 149 (142 -156) | 1,950 | 2,250 | 2,550 | 3,000 |
| | Large | 161 (151- 170) | 2,100 | 2,400 | 2,750 | 3,200 |
| 5'9" | Small | 145(140- 150) | 1,900 | 2,200 | 2,450 | 2,900 |
| | Medium | 153 (146 -160) | 2,000 | 2,300 | 2,600 | 3,050 |
| | Large | 165 (155- 174) | 2,150 | 2,500 | 2,800 | 3,300 |
| 5'10" | Small | 149 (144- 154) | 1,950 | 2,250 | 2,550 | 3,000 |
| | Medium | 158 (150 -165) | 2,050 | 2,350 | 2,700 | 3,150 |
| | Large | 169 (159- 179) | 2,200 | 2,500 | 2,850 | 3,400 |
| 5'11" | Small | 153 (148- 158) | 2,000 | 2,300 | 2,600 | 3,050 |
| | Medium | 162 (154 -170) | 2,100 | 2,450 | 2,750 | 3,250 |
| | Large | 174 (164- 184) | 2,250 | 2,600 | 2,850 | 3,500 |

**Table: 6.4. Desirable weights and calorie levels for women**

| Height without Shoes* | Frame Size | Desirable Weight (pound) | Very Light (Calorie) | Light (Calorie) | Moderate (Calorie) | Heavy (Calorie) |
|---|---|---|---|---|---|---|
| 5'0" | Small | 106 (102- 110) | 1,400 | 1,600 | 1,800 | 2,100 |
| | Medium | 113 (107 -119) | 1,450 | 1,700 | 1,900 | 2,250 |
| | Large | 123 (115- 131) | 1,600 | 1,850 | 2,100 | 2,450 |
| 5'1" | Small | 109 (105- 113) | 1,400 | 1,650 | 1,850 | 2,200 |
| | Medium | 116 (110 -122) | 1,500 | 1,750 | 1,950 | 2,300 |
| | Large | 126 (118- 134) | 1,650 | 1,900 | 2,150 | 2,500 |
| 5'2" | Small | 112 (108- 116) | 1,450 | 1,700 | 1,900 | 2,250 |
| | Medium | 119 (113 -126) | 1,550 | 1,800 | 2,000 | 2,400 |
| | Large | 129 (121- 138) | 1,700 | 1,950 | 2,200 | 2,600 |
| 5'3" | Small | 115 (111- 119) | 1,500 | 1,750 | 1,950 | 2,300 |
| | Medium | 123 (116 -130) | 1,600 | 1,850 | 2,100 | 2,450 |
| | Large | 133 (125- 142) | 1,750 | 2,000 | 2,250 | 2,650 |
| 5'4" | Small | 118 (114- 123) | 1,550 | 1,750 | 2,000 | 2,350 |
| | Medium | 127 (120 -135) | 1,650 | 1,900 | 2,150 | 2,550 |
| | Large | 137 (129- 146) | 1,800 | 2,050 | 2,350 | 2,750 |
| 5'5" | Small | 122 (118- 127) | 1,600 | 1,850 | 2,050 | 2,450 |
| | Medium | 131 (124 -139) | 1,700 | 1,950 | 2,250 | 2,600 |
| | Large | 141 (133- 150) | 1,850 | 2,100 | 2,400 | 2,800 |

| Height without Shoes* | Frame Size | Desirable Weight (pound) | Very Light (Calorie) | Light (Calorie) | Moderate (Calorie) | Heavy (Calorie) |
|---|---|---|---|---|---|---|
| 5’6” | Small | 126 (122- 131) | 1,650 | 1,900 | 2,150 | 2,500 |
| | Medium | 135 (128 -143) | 1,750 | 2,050 | 2,300 | 2,700 |
| | Large | 145 (137- 154) | 1,900 | 2,200 | 2,450 | 2,900 |
| 5’7” | Small | 130 (126- 135) | 1,700 | 1,950 | 2,200 | 2,600 |
| | Medium | 139 (132 -147) | 1,800 | 2,100 | 2,350 | 2,800 |
| | Large | 149 (141- 158) | 1,950 | 2,250 | 2,550 | 3,000 |
| 5’8” | Small | 135 (130- 140) | 1,750 | 2,050 | 2,300 | 2,700 |
| | Medium | 143 (136 -151) | 1,850 | 2,150 | 2,450 | 2,850 |
| | Large | 154 (145 -163) | 2,000 | 2,300 | 2,600 | 3,100 |
| 5’9” | Small | 139 (134- 144) | 1,800 | 2,100 | 2,350 | 2,800 |
| | Medium | 147 (140 -155) | 1,900 | 2,200 | 2,500 | 2,950 |
| | Large | 158 (149- 168) | 2,050 | 2,350 | 2,700 | 3,150 |
| 5’10” | Small | 143 (138- 148) | 1,850 | 2,150 | 2,450 | 2,850 |
| | Medium | 151 (144 -159) | 1,950 | 2,250 | 2,550 | 3,000 |
| | Large | 163 (153- 173) | 2,100 | 2,450 | 2,750 | 3,250 |

## 6.5 Intake of Excessive Iron

Too much iron can make an individual old by fostering free radical attacks on cells. Supplements of iron should be avoided unless they are taken on the advice of a physician.

Excess iron can be very dangerous, because it facilitates free radical damage to cells. For example, iron helps change benign LDL cholesterol into toxic type that wrecks arteries and makes heart fail. Intake of excess iron can be avoided by:

- Cutting down on animal food. The heme iron in meat is absorbed more readily than the non-heme iron in vegetables such as beans and cereals. Red meat is particularly bad, since iron and red meat combination produce peroxides and free radicals.
- Consume food and beverages such as tea, red wine and high fibre bran and beans that tend to block absorption of iron.
- Do not take iron-fortified cereals.
- One may donate blood, 2-3 times a year to deplete unwanted iron store.
- Children and childbearing women need iron supplements. This should be taken only on the advice of one's physician.

## 6.6 Keeping Physically Fit

Physical fitness plays a vital role in delaying aging and prolonging life. However, there are some people who believe in the following two things:

- If an individual is healthy, one does not need to exercise.

- If an individual is sick, one should not exercise.

It goes beyond doubt that the above points are not correct. In fact exercise has a marked effect on improving the immune system (Tomasi et al, J Clin. Immunol, 1982, **2**, 173-178; Soppi et al., J. Clin. Lab. Immunol., 1982, **8**, 43-46; Hanson et al., Clin. Soc., 1981, **60**, 225-228). On the basis of various studies, it has been found that exercising produces a higher number of white blood cells, especially the granulocytes that are needed to ward off or fight off infections or tumors. The higher count remained elevated for 40-45 minutes after the exercise. The lymphocytes count was also elevated in people who exercise. This elevation was also transient and returned to normal after the exercise. In a number of studies in animals, it has been shown that exercising regularly can inhibit cancer growth (Gershbein, L. L. et al., Oncology, 1974, **30**, 429) A number of studies on human beings show that increased physical activity promotes health with less disease in general and a longer life (E. Paffenberger, NEJM, 1986, **314**, 605-613)

Exercising has a tremendously life affirming and stress reducing effect. Besides this, following are some more advantages of exercising:

- It helps reduce all cancers by enhancing the immune function.
- Exercise helps to increase the levels of natural killer cells; the activity of these cells also increases with regular exercising.
- It reduces the risk of colorectal cancer by promoting bowel contraction. Increased contraction speeds waste products through the intestines, thereby decreasing the chance for

carcinogens and the colorectum lining to come into contact. It has been found that there is 25-50% lower incidence of colon cancer among those people who exercise at moderate to high levels, as compared with people who do not exercise at all.

- It helps to reduce the risk of prostrate cancer, possibly by lowering the testosterone levels. This has been supported by a number of studies. It is known that this disease occurs as a result of the testes producing excess levels of the male hormone 'testosterone'.
- It helps to reduce the risk of breast cancer, uterine cancer and ovarian cancer, possibly by lowering the female hormone 'estrogen'. It is known that higher levels of estrogen can stimulate abnormal cell growth in each of the above organs, leading to cancer. Exercising or any other physical activity not only alters the hormone ratio favorably but also improves body fat distribution. It has been found that there is higher incidence of uterine cancer amongst women who are heavy in the upper and mid body. On the whole, exercising also keeps a control on the individual's weight.
- Regular exercise improves sleep, reduces headaches, creates a feeling of well-being and increases concentration and stamina. Endorphins are released into the brain during exercise; these chemicals promote a sense of happiness and positivity.
- Exercise is an effective tool in the fight against depressors and a vital move in the preparation for a relaxed life.

- It helps to keep the heart healthy, thereby lowering the risks (like increasing level of HDL (good) cholesterol, decreasing the level of LDL (bad) cholesterol, lowering triglyceride level, lowering blood pressure; all this helps in preventing heart attack and stroke.
- It also decreases the concentration of sugar (glucose) in the body making the cells in the body more sensitive to insulin. This is particularly useful for management of diabetes.
- Exercise also helps in reduction and management of stress.

On the basis of the above it can be stated that exercise plays a major role in preventing aging so that one can live a long and happy life.

The question that arises is 'what form of exercise is the best?' most experts advice some form of non-competitive exercise, like swimming, weight training or walking. It is best to consult one's doctor and seek advice on which form of exercise is best.

Generally speaking exercises are of two types:

**Aerobic exercise:**

It uses large group of muscles and can be continued for a long period of time. Some examples are walking, jogging, swimming, cycling etc. Aerobic exercise makes the body use oxygen present in air effectively and gives maximum benefit to the heart, lungs and the circulatory system.

**Anaerobic exercise:**

It builds muscles strength, muscle endurance and bone density. Examples include weight lifting, wrestling etc. In such exercises, the body does not get time to use oxygen efficiently and are harmful for people with high blood pressure.

Benefits of exercising are immense. Although they cannot be measured with a scale, a healthy body instills a sense of pleasure, vitality and well-being. Following are given some of the most convenient forms of exercises, which are very helpful for slowing down aging and prolonging, an individual's life span.

**(i) Brisk Walking**

Brisk walking improves muscle condition, blood circulation and posture. All one needs is a good pair of shoes (strong and light weight) and a waterproof jacket. Start by walking for 30 minutes a day. Walk fast enough to make oneself a little out of breath.

After a week, increase the time of walking to about 45 minutes and after 2-3 weeks make it 60 minutes. After 4-6 weeks of brisk walking one will sleep better, the concentration will be sharper and the individual will feel emotionally balanced. By getting into the habit of walking briskly every day, one will be rewarded with a fit body, glowing skin and a sense of well-being.

**(ii) Running**

Running is the most satisfying form of aerobic exercise for most of the persons. One should be dressed as discussed in brisk walking. Before starting, it is important to check one's fitness. This can be easily done by walking 5 km's in 30 minutes. If one does not feel any nausea or dizziness, one is fit to start the running exercise.

The following program can be followed:

*First week*:

Walk briskly for 1.5 km's occasionally doing a jog during walking, walk at a steady pace. One should not force one self to do so.

*Second week*:

Walk/Jog for 1.5 km's alternating about 100 strides of each at a stretch.

*Third week*:

Repeat the walk/jog as in second week with jogging intervals to 150 strides with 100 strides of walking in between.

*Fourth week:*

Jog for a while at a speed, which is most comfortable.

*Fifth week:*

Run 1.5 km's in less than 10 minutes.

*Sixth week:*

Jog/Run for 3 km's or more everyday.

By the end of the sixth week, an individual's stamina will be increased.

To get the benefits, run for at least 30 minutes a day. One will find that running has become addictive.

It is important to cool properly after a run. It can be done by walking for 5-10 minutes after every run.

**(iii) Deep breathing exercise**

The air which is to breathe must be the purest available. Following steps are followed:

(a) Sit straight with your back straight. Inhale slowly through nose. Make sure the stomach is expanding as lungs get filled with air. While inhaling, the abdomen must be relaxed.

(b) After taking a full breath, inhale some more air.

(c) Hold breath for 3-4 seconds.

(d) Expel the air through mouth. Also use stomach muscles to squeeze all the air. Try to squeeze some more air.

(e) Pause for a second with empty lungs.

(f) Inhale once more. Repeat the process of inhalation and exhalation three times.

(g) Do this exercise at least 3-4 times a day.

Deep breathing exercises can be done during the morning walk also.

**(iv) Stretching exercise**

A number of stretching exercises can be performed. Some of these are:

**Exercise 1: Rolling Shoulders**

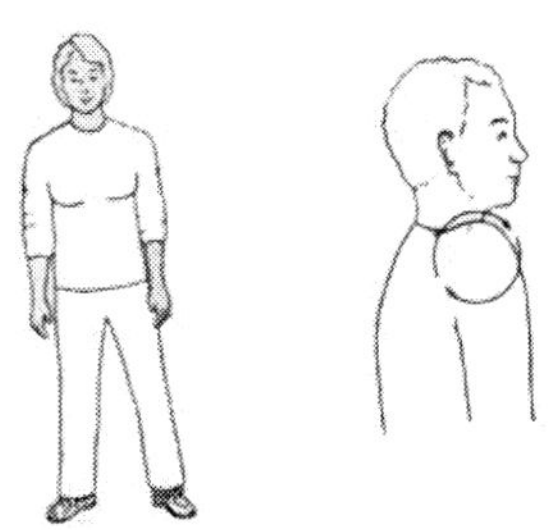

**Fig. 6.1. Rolling Shoulders**

Stand in a relaxed manner (Fig. 6.1(a)) keeping the feet wide apart and the arms hanging loosely. Breathe normally. Slowly start shrugging and rolling both shoulders at the same time, circling them in clockwise direction (Fig. 6.1(b))(shoulder would move forward and upwards the ears and then back around and down to the position from which you started). Note that the shoulders rotate in a full circle.

**Exercise 2: Swinging the Arms**

Stand in a relaxed position as in exercise 1. Keeping the right hand relaxed, slowly bringing it up in front of you (Fig. 6.2) and then back around to its starting position after completing a circle. Repeat the exercise two more times. Then exercise with the left arm in the same way. Again repeat the circle in the opposite direction first by right hand and then by the left hand (3 times with each hand).

Finally repeat the circle (Fig. 6.2) swinging the arm with both hands together in both directions (3 times in each direction). The only precaution is to do it slowly and easily.

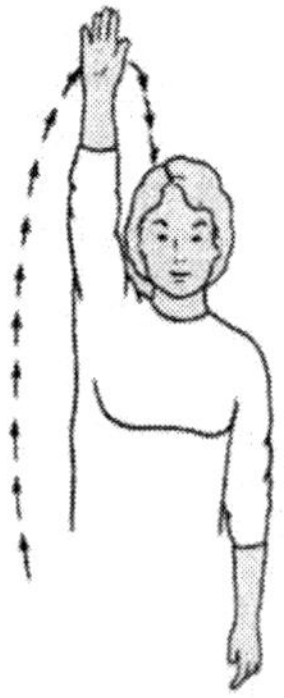

**Fig. 6.2. Swinging the Arms**

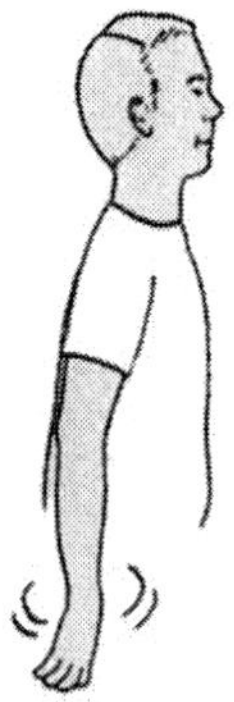

**Fig. 6.3. Swinging the fists**

**Exercise 3: Swinging the Fist**

Stand in relaxed position (as in exercise 1). Keep the right hand relaxed. Slowly swing only the fist first in clockwise direction (3 times). Repeat with fist of the left then in anti-clockwise direction (3 times). Repeat with fist of the left hand (3 times swing in a circle in both the directions). Finally, swing both fists (3 times each in both directions) (Fig. 6.3).

**Exercise 4: Stretching the Upper Body**

Stand in relaxed manner (as in exercise 1). Take both the arm backwards (keeping the arms straight). The arms be taken up as far as possible without feeling any pain (Fig. 6.4(a)). After your arms have reached maximum extension, bring both arms in the original position. Take both the arms forward (in front of you), bend the elbows and bring the hands up, so that the finger touch the shoulders. This will leave the upper arm parallel to the ground (Fig. 6.4(b)).

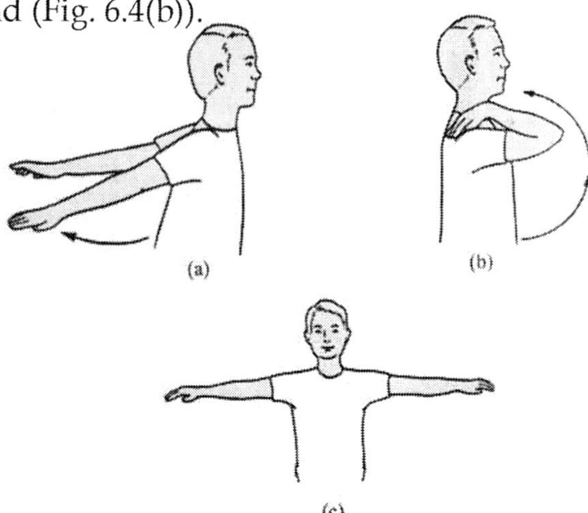


**Fig. 6.4. Stretching the Upper Body**

Finally straighten bothe the arms to the side so that the body is in T-shape (Fig. 6.4(c)). Lower the arms and hands to the side and return to the original starting position. Repeat the total series three times.

**Exercise 5: Twisting the Torso**

Stand in a relaxed manner (as in exercise 1). Raise both the arms out in front of you until they are parallel to the

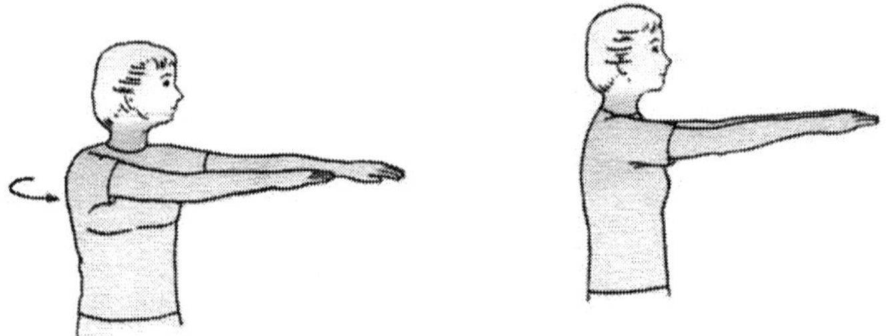

(a) (b)

**Fig. 6.5. Twisting the Torso**

ground. The fingers should be pointing straight ahead (Fig. 6.5(a)). Now slowly twist the torso to the left (Fig. 6.5(b)) (keeping the back straight) without moving the feet, legs or hips. Please understand that you want to twist the upper body only. The movement should extend from your head to your waist.

Twist as far as possible to the left and then without pausing swing back to the right. Do not over do the stretch. Go only to the extent you can comfortably do. Twist the torso to the left and then to the right in a continuous process without waiting or pausing at any intermediate position. Two complete left-right swings are sufficient.

**Exercise 6: Twisting the Neck**

The exercise should be done slowly and as gently as possible.

Stand in a relaxed manner (as in exercise 1). Turn the head to the left as far as possible (without moving the shoulder or torso) (Fig. 6.6(a)) and then return to the starting position. Next turn the head to the right as much as possible (Fig. 6.6(b)) and then return to the starting position. Finally, let the head slump forward (very slowly) so that the chin is toward the chest (Fig. 6.6(c)).

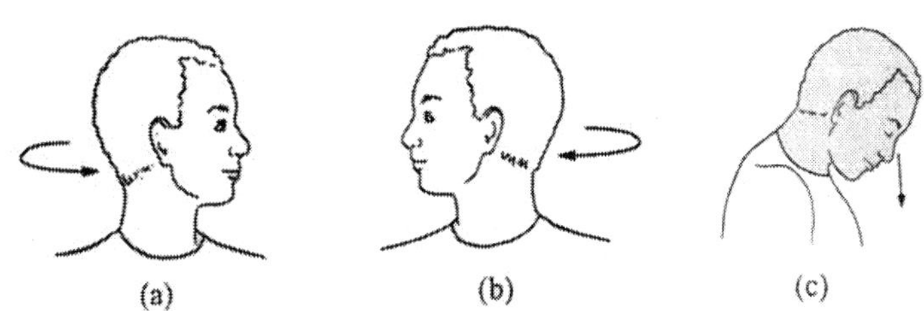


**Fig. 6.6. Twisting the Neck**

Then lift the head back and return to the starting position. In the total exercise, movements should be slow and there should be no jerk or thrust on the head. Repeat the total process of turning your head to the left, right, down and back three times. The idea of this exercise is to stretch your neck very lightly. Repeat the total exercise thrice.

**Exercise 7: Stretching the Arms**

Stand in a relaxed manner (as in exercise 1). Lift both hands to the middle of your chest. interwine the fingers so that the palms face each other (Fig. 6.7(a)). Keeping the finger inter wined and palms facing each other, slowly straighten the arms in a straight position, reaching towards the ceiling or sky as far as you can comfortably do (Fig. 6.7(b)). Finally roll the palms outwards (without unwinding the fingers) and continue rotating the wrist and forearms until the palms face upwards (Fig. 6.7(c)). In the final phase of exercise you should feel the stretch in the wrist and forearm. Hold this position for a few seconds and then rotate the wrist and forearm back and lower the arms to the middle of the breast. Do the series of exercise twice.

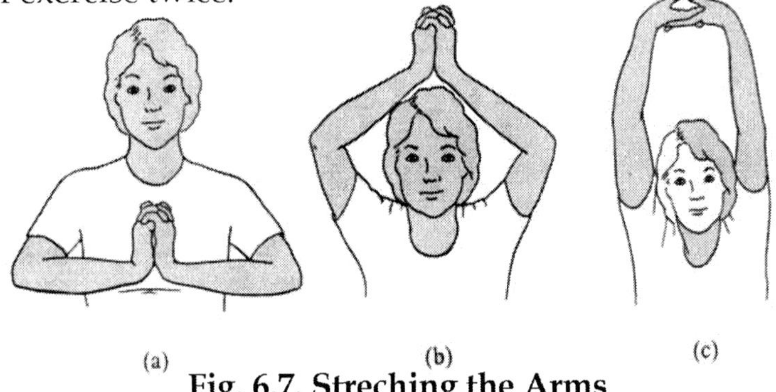


**Fig. 6.7. Streching the Arms**

**Exercise 8: Streching the Legs**

Stand in a relaxed manner (as in exercise 1). Keeping the feet close to each other (Fig. 6.8(a)). Raise yourself up on your toes as far as you can (Fig. 6.8(b)). Then lower yourself back on your heels (Fig. 6.8(a)). Finally lift your toes up off the ground (Fig. 6.8(c)). Repeat the total steps five times.

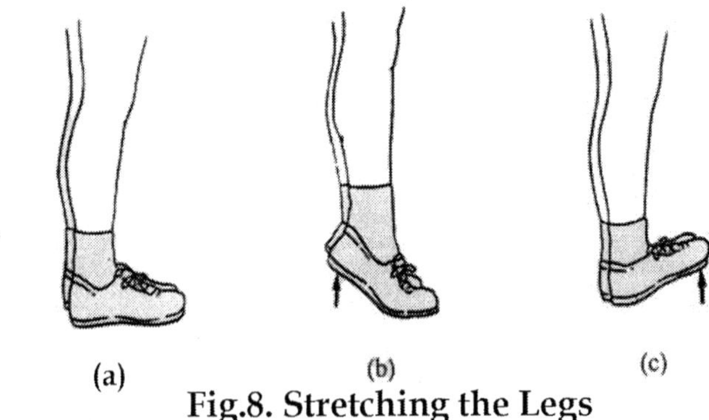


**Fig.8. Stretching the Legs**

**Exercise 9: Stretching the Back**

Start in the position as shown in Fig. 6.9(a) with the hands and knees on the floor and the back parallel to the floor. Lower the head gently and take (or stretch) the back upwards (as much as possible) (Fig. 6.9(b)). Then return the head and back to their original positions. Repeat twice.

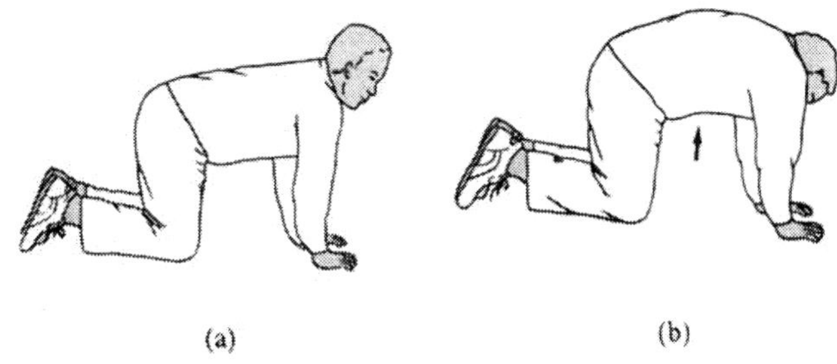

(a) (b)

**Fig. 6.9. Stretching the Back**

**Exercise 10: Twisting the Legs**

Stand in a relaxed manner (as in exercise 1). Put both the hands on the waist. Now slowly twist the body (the lower portion up to the waist) in clockwise direction. After taking five turns, twist the body in anticlockwise direction five times. Repeat the total exercise three times completing five turns in each direction.

The number of exercises suggested are sufficient for most of the people. The routine for the stretching exercise is simple, quick and effective. The only thing is to do them slowly and staying relaxed. This set of exercise will take about 15 minutes.

**(v) Yoga**

Yogic exercises are the best for keeping healthy and active. People doing yogic exercises can really delay aging and lead a healthy, long and meaningful life. A Yoga expert should be consulted for doing Yoga in the correct way.

## 6.7 Stress Versus Aging

It has been suggested that physical factors such as

stress, influence a person's immune system response and so he becomes susceptible to infectious diseases, cancer, heart ailments etc. Factors like stress and emotions are known to worsen some common types of headaches, other syndromes and irritable bowel movement. Stress also affects many diseases including asthma, hypertension, ulcers, diabetes, arthritis and other autoimmune disease.

What is stress? When we are tensed, agitated and irritable, we say that we have symptoms of stress. In fact, stress can be defined as our mental, emotional and physical response to the irritants, challenges and threats. one may feel stressed due to loss of car keys, waiting for a long time for an appointment or getting late, while others may not be stressed under these conditions. Stress cannot be measured with an instrument like blood pressure or cholesterol level in blood. Stress can only be felt.

If a person is under stress for a considerable length of time, he/she will show premature aging. In view of this, it is essential to find out the cause of stress in life and one should try to remove it. It is best to keep smiling in stressful situations.

On being confronted with a situation, a person may tend to be under stress. In such a situation, the nervous system and hormones from the adrenal gland (mainly adrenaline) automatically trigger a number of physical changes in order to facilitate the body's capacity to fight or face stress. In such a situation, the heart rate and blood pressure may increase, and the muscles may be tensed up. These physical adaptations in response to stress are observable and established.

It has been established that people suffering from heart disease suffer from heart pain when they are stressed. In fact, due to stress, there is rapid increase of heart rate and blood pressure, which in turn, generates a greater demand for oxygen by the heart and brings about chest pain (attack of angina pectoris).

Due to stress there is an increased secretion of hormone and intensified blood circulation. The combination of the two situations during stress response can damage the lining of the arteries. The result is that arterial walls may harden or thicken and become more susceptible to the build up of plaque. Thus, the flow of blood is impaired leading to heart attack. Also, there is an increased likelihod of blood clotting, blockage of the artery resulting in a heart attack. On the basis of several studies it has been found that:

(a) Life of a person suffering from angina is at the mercy of a person who chooses to upset him and increase his stress.

(b) The risk of a heart attack increase about 14 times on the day of the death of a close relative or a friend.

(c) Risk for having a heart attack is more than doubled during first two hours of an episode of anger.

(d) The stress created by earthquake or war sharply increases the death rate due to sudden cardiac arrests.

It is thus concluded that stress can contribute to the risk of heart attacks. It is not conclusively established that stress can cause heart disease. We can, however, say that stress accelerates certain heart conditions.

How much a person gets affected by stress depends on his personality. One type of person (say type A) is impatient, easily provoked to hostility, irritating and work obsessed. The other type, say B is more relaxed, always smiling, does not work in a hurry and is satisfied with the degree of success. Type B can still be achievement oriented but are not as type A, who wants to accomplish results in a short span of time. The traits in type A people may be dangerous to ones health. According to studies, type A people have double the risk of developing coronary heart disease compared to type B.

Since stress is a risk factor for heart disease, it is responsible to conclude that jobs with the highest stress have highest mortality rates. This is not true, because the response to stressful situations vary with different people. We know that some people enjoy working under stress.

**Managing Stress**

Stress is an unavoidable part of life. The most important things is to learn to live with it and also to learn about its management. The basic principles of stress management are:

(i) To recognize when you are feeling overstressed.

(ii) To identify the cause of stress in your life.

(iii) To minimize the effects of stress on your mind and body.

**Recognizing when you feel overstressed**

This important step in the management of stress is not as easy as it sounds. The best way to recognize overstress is to note any of the common symptoms listed in Table 6.5.

**Table: 6.5. Symtoms of Stress**

| | |
|---|---|
| Increase in heart beats | Anxiety |
| Cold hands | Irritability |
| Feeling of fatigue | Impatience |
| Dry mouth | Grinding teeth |
| Difficulty in breathing | Too much eating |
| Tight facial muscles | Too much drinking |
| Sudden sweating | Chain smoking |
| Face turning red | Nail biting |
| Headache | Constant picking at face |
| Upset stomach | Fiddling with, twisting or |
| Sudden anger | Pulling out hair |
| Talking too much | Inability to express |
| Sudden tears without any cause | Depression |

In case you experience at least three of the symptoms (Table 6.5), you may be experiencing too much stress. It should be kept in mind that some of the symptoms may be due to some other conditions other than stress. In such a situation, consult your doctor.

## Identifying the cause of stress in you life

Once you recognize that you are under stress, keep dialy record of when and why you feel stressed. See if there is any pattern. By careful analysis you will be able to identify the cause of stress in your life.

Couple of times each day for a week check the signs of stress in you and note the time and cause of each episode. Stressful events may include sudden anger over a trivial matter (such as a car ahead of you waiting too long after the light has turned green, annoyance for being kept waiting for an appointment or an exchange of words with someone). Each time you feel tense, try to analyze why. It may be a specific event. Keep a record for about a week then carefully analyse as to what caused stress in your life.

In order to deal with stress, first modify as many situations as possible that create stress in your life, e.g., if you get stressed for being late for keeping an appointment due to too much traffic, you may either try to change the route where there is less traffic or start early in order to reach in time. Alternatively, you may keep the time of appointment at an hour when there is less traffic jams. Next, think about the conditions on which you have no control. Try to rethink your mental attitude towards those conditions you cannot change. If you believe in a thing that cannot be cured must be (or has to be) endured, there will be no difficulty in learning to live with what you cannot change. In other words, you may not feel stressed.

As seen above, you have no control over the traffic jam and hence no control on the time you would take to reach for the appointment. Think, there is no point in getting angry or stressed. Keep your cool and use one of the relaxation techniques. Also think why you become tense. Is it because you are blocked by a traffic jam or are late for the appointment or you did not start early. Understanding the reason will make you less emotional or stressed. Finally, think of alternatives to avoid such an experience again.

**Minimizing the effect of stress on the mind and body**

The most effective means of moderating stress and hence minimizing its effect on the body and mind is exercising. So, a regular exercise programme will help in the management of stress. For a fitness programme. (see section 6.5) If you are not exercising, start doing it today itself. Do not postpone it for some other day. It is found that most of the people who are stressed notice that their muscles tend to stiffen and become tense. For this, slow stretching exercise brings the tightness of the muscles to normal state and promotes relaxing.

Relaxing is another critical factor for minimizing the effects of stress on your mind and body. It is possible to relax in the most stressful situations. This can be achieved by deep breathing.

**Deep breathing exercise**

This exercise should be performed in the following steps:

(i) Sit with the back straight. Inhale slowly through the nose. Make sure that the stomach is expanding as the lungs get filled. While inhaling the abdomen must be relaxed.

(ii) When you think you have taken a fully breath, try to inhale a little more air.

(iii) Hold your breath for 3-4 seconds.

(iv) Exhale the air through the mouth. Also use the stomach muscles to squeeze all the air you can. Try to squeeze out just a little bit more.

(v) With your lungs empty, pause for a second.

(vi) Begin inhaling and exhaling (three times).

(vii) Do this deep breathing exercise 3-4 times a day especially when you feel stressed.

**Mental focus**

(i) Select a number, a name or a word (whatever you like).

(ii) Stretch out on a bed or lie on the floor. Feel comfortable and close your eyes.

(iii) Relax all the muscles. Starting from the toes and proceed upwards checking muscles of the feet, ankles, shins, thighs, stomach, back, chest, shoulders, neck, and face. Ensure that all muscles are relaxed. When you reach the scalp, silently repeat to yourself (without speaking loud) the number or name or word you have selected. Say it over and over again (10-15 times) in you mind, keeping the eyes closed and muscles relaxed throughout. You feel relaxed if you focus on the word.

**Reduce stress whenever you can**

If you are stressful or you think that you have too much stress, you can reduce stresss by following some of these:

(a) Drive slowly.

(b) Walk slowly.

(c) Take more time to comeplete any task.

(d) Remember to relax when you are confronted to any stressful situation.

(e) If you have to wait for meeting or appointments use the time for reading a magazine or newspaper.

(f) Do not set objectives that are difficult to meet.

(g) Think positively.

(h) Enjoy the company of friends.

(i) Do not be aggressive or passive to get what you want. In fact be assertive.

(j) Minimize crisis situations by keeping yourself well organized.

(k) Find time for resting.

(l) Spend time on your hobbies. If you do not have any hobbies, find or cultivate some, e.g. Listening to music or watching a movie.

**Miscellaneous relaxation techniques**

Following are some simple techniques by which you can reduce the level fo stress or even eliminate stress in you life.

1. Reduce intake of coffee. Studies how that people who drink too much coffee or beverages containing coffeine while working experience stress.
2. Avoid dependence on alcohol, drugs or nicotine. These are not stress relievers but are stress intensifiers.
3. Take a warm shower.
4. Reduce the intake of sugar, too much of it can increase stress.
5. Keep smiling. respond to any stressful situation smilingly.
6. When working concentrate only on work.
7. Crying releases anxiety. If you are stressed due to some event try to cry. Tears will reduce the stress.
8. Perform any task assigned to you to the best of your capability. Striving for unattainable perfection pronounces stress.
9. Do meditation to reduce or even eliminate stress.

Management of stress is the key to improving your outlook of life and to have closer relations with your friends, associates and loved ones. Stress management gives benefits, which go beyond the benefits of removing a risk factor of heart disease from your life.

(a) Whenever you are stressed, smile at the reason, which has made you stressed.

(b) When you are getting angry ask yourself a question "Is the incident on which you are getting angry important"? If the answer is yes, ask the second question "Is the anger justified"? Again if the answer is yes, ask the final question, "Do I have an effective response"? If you have an effective response, to the situation act on it. If there is no response, which means that your anger won't change the situation. By reasoning to yourself in this way, you can manage or overcome your anger.

(c) Do not get angry or stressed if the answer to your question is no. You should analyze in your mind why it is so. This way you will be able to manage your stress.

# 7

# AGE PROTECTORS

Though aging is a natural phenomenon, but its onset can be considerable delayed. A very important aspect is to protect the body from Life-Robbing Diseases. Some of such diseases along with strategies to prevent them are given below.

## 7.1 Arthritis

Though arthritis is beloved to be the disease of the elderly, it usually begins fairly early in life. The best is to follow some very effective techniques for stopping arthritis even before it strikes. Although there are more than 100 kinds of arthritis, the most common are oesteoarthritis and rheumatoid arthritis. When one gets arthritis the joints natural movements get rough and creaky. The lubrication declines and the cartilage gradually wears away. Instead of sliding smoothly, the bones begin to grate. This is what causes pain, stifness, inflammation and other arthritis symptoms. The pain caused by arthritis can be eased by:

(i) Applying heat by using a heating pad or hot pack in a towel 3 times a day for 20 minutes each times is helpful.

(ii) Applying cold bath, chilling the joint helps constrict blood vessels.

(iii) Applying some commonly available creams. One such cream, which is effective is made from Linseed oil, menthol and camphor.

## Prevention of Arthritis

### (i) Use Correct Posture

Bad posture puts lots of pressure on various joints, causing bone and cartilage to wear away in certain spots and can cause pain. One should make sure that one is sitting or standing straight. While reading do not put unnecessary pressure on your neck and lower back; this could lead to problems at a subsequent stage. The basic idea is to sit and stand in such a way that the bones are evenly balanced, rather than veering off at odd angles. The way one walks can be as good or bad in a similar way as one stands. Waking should not cause pressure on vulnerable joints.

### (ii) Consume Balanced Diet

One should eat a balanced diet containing plenty of vegetables, fruits and grains and take in only moderate amounts of sugar, salt, fat, cholesterol and alcohol. Follow the well known saying, 'Eat right and live longer.' To combat the free radicals, it is necessary to get more of antioxidant nutrients, such as vitamins C and E in the diet.

### (iii) Sleep in a Natural Way

Avoid using pillows for propping up the head when sleeping; this can put unnecessary stress on a number of joints. The best is to sleep in natural posture, i.e., lying on the back or side and keeping neck in line with the back, with arms and legs in a soft, relaxed position; the elbows, wrists, knees and ankles can be bent very slightly. This way of sleeping puts least possible stress and is also smoothing in case there is a flare of arthritis.

**(iv) Exercising**

Though osteoarthritis is considered to be problem of the bones, it often begins in the muscles. So it is very important to keep the muscles strong. The programme of exercising must be decided in consultation with your physician. Generally speaking, the programme should include involvement of knee and hip, toes, shoulder, fingers, back, ankles.

## 7.2 Cancer

Cancer is the most dreadful of all diseases and is believed to be the second most common cause of death. It comprises of a group of 120-150 diseases which can either arise within or outside the body. However, all cancers have a characteristic, i.e., uncontrolled cell growth. It normally develops cell by cell, often taking years to cause problems.

**Who is at higher risk factor for development of cancer.**

A person who is accustomed to taking meat (particularly red meat), who is obese, smoker, takes alcohol and is exposed to radiation and comes in contact (as inhales) with carsogenic chemicals like benene, aniline etc. and has a personal history or family history or a family member having cancer and does little exercise and leads a stressful life belongs to the high-risk category (which may or may not develop cancer). In fact all the factors mentioned above are responsible for the development of cancer. It is believed that passive smokers (people who inhale smoke emitted by smokers) are at greater risk for the development of cancer.

## Cancer Prevention Programme

Following are given some of the important guidelines—suggestions which will not only reduce the risk of new cancers cases, but will also help in checking the cancer to spread.

(i) **Nutrition.** Consume a low animal fat and low cholestrol diet. It is best to take vegetarian diet. People who are vegetarian and consume nutritious diet have very low chances of developing cancer, heart disease, blood pressure and diabetes. For a vegetarian diet, it is best to combine legumes (lentils, peas, dried beans) which are low in amino acid methionine and whole grain (e.g., rice, wheat, corn, oats, etc.) which are low in amino acid lysine. Thus a combination of a legume and a grain in a vegetarian diet can provide appropriate amount of amino acid or complete proteins. In order to ensure intake of all the essential amino acids, the vegetarian diet should include non-fat diary products like skimmed or low fat milk, non-fat yogurt, cheese and egg whites. The vegetarian diet should supply nutrients like vitamin B12 iron, calcium, vitamin D, zinc.

Following tables given the various nutrients and their sources:

| Nutrients | Plants Source |
|---|---|
| Vitamin B12 | Some cereals (like maze), fortified soy milk, yogurt, cheese, eggs |
| Iron | Dried beans, whole grains, dark green leafy vegetables, dried fruits, prune juice, whole wheat bread.<br>Absorption of iron is increased by |

| | |
|---|---|
| | Vitamin C found in cirtrus fruits and juices, tomatoes, strawberries, broccoli, peppers, dark green leafy vegetables, potatoes with skin. |
| Calcium | Tofu (Prepared with calcium), broccoli, seeds, nuts, spinach, turnip, legumes (beans and peas) |
| Vitamin D | Milk fortified with Vitamin D, Cod liver oil |
| Zinc | Whole grains (especially the germ and bran proteins), whole wheat bread, legumes, nuts and tofu. |

(ii) **Tabacco.** Do not start smoking just for the heck of it. It is not fashionable to smoke

- If you have a habit of smoking, quit it.
- As a non-smoker do not become a passive smoker (inhaling smoke emitted by smokers)
- As a non-smoker, insist that smoking is not allowed in public or work related areas.
- Do not chew or snuff tabacco.

(iii) **Alcohol**

- If you do not drink, do not start it.
- Abstain from alcohol consumption or reduce to a minimum (one drink per week)
- Consumption of even modest amout of alcohol in a week is a risk factor for breast cancer and other cancers.

(iv) **Radiation**

- Avoid exposure to ionizing radiation. e.g. exposure to x-ray for diagnostic purposes. Diagnosis should only be done on strict advice of a physician.
- Avoid ultravoilet light (as emitted by Sun) particularly at noon time (sunlight causes cancer of the skin).
- Avoid sun tanning parlours.

(v) **Occupational Risk**

- Exposure to a number of industries that manufacture dyes, chemicals, rubber, paint, electroplating, or poisons gases, nickel, plastic and a large number of other industries which use chemicals, may cause cancer of various types. Workers in these industries should take appropriate precaution.
- Avoid prolonged exposure to household cleaning fluids, solvents, paint thinners, pesticides, fungicides, etc.
- Avoid exposure to electromagnetic radiation for a long time.

(vi) **Sexual Behaviour**

- Practice safe sex.
- Avoid multiple sex partners. If necessary, use condoms to reduce the risk of sexually transmitted virus which can cause cancer.
- Women having extra marital relations (sex) should insist that the male partner use a condom.
- Avoid use of illicit drugs.

(vii) **Stress**

- Reduce stress in your life for details (see page 96).

(viii) **Obesity**

- Avoid over eating.
- Eat a well-balanced diet.
- Follow a regular exercise programme (see page 83).

## 7.3 Heart Disease

Heart disease is the most common cause of death all over the world. It accounts for more deaths than all other diseases combined together. It is estimated that about 95% of all heart attacks happen to people over 40 years of age. However, there are some cases reported in which very young people aged 20-30 years also suffer heart attacks. Heart disease is an entirely consequence of the way we live.

### Who is at higher risk for heart disease

Certain risk factors for heart disease which cannot be controlled are age, gender and genetic factors. There are other risk factors which can be controlled. These include, smoking, high blood pressure, high cholesterol levels (particularly higher level of LDL), Diabetes mellitus, obesity. People who do not keep a check on the factors (given above) which can be controlled have higher risk of heart ailments. In addition, people who are physically inactive, consume alcohol and are non-vegetarians (consumes red meat) and are stressed have additional risk for development of heart disease.

## Prevention of Heart Disease

The only way to prevent the heart disease is to keep a check on the risk factors which are responsible for heart attacks. In other words, the heart must be kept healthy and in good shape. Following are given some of the important guidelines/suggestions to keep the heart healthy.

### (i) Smoking

The advice given by experts is very clear. "If you smoke, stop it; if you don't smoke don't start it". Some people stop smoking on the advice of doctors when they have a life threatening disease (for example cardiovascular disease or cancer). The advice of the doctor is very specific "If you want to live, stop smoking". There are other categories of people who stop smoking after they have understood the following threats caused by smoking:

- Smokers are twice as much likely to have a heart attack then non-smokers.
- Sudden cardiac death is three to four times more common in smokers than in non-smokers.
- Smoking is responsible for about 90% of all cases of lung cancer.
- Smoking is responsible for about 30% of all cancer deaths.
- Smoking is responsible for about 20% of all deaths of coronary heart disease.
- In case of smokers, there is increased risk for stroke, chronic bronchitis, sexual impotence.
- A cardiovascular disease (peripheral vascular disease) in which the vessels carrying blood to the

arms or legs are narrowed is exclusively prevalent in smokers.

- Smoking harms not only the smokers, but also other people who inhale the secondary smoke exhaled by the smokers. Such people are known as passive smokers.
- The children living in homes where parent(s) smoke and even the unborn child in a mother's womb are all adversely effected by second hand or secondary smoke.
- Teenagers whose parent(s) smoke are more likely to acquire the habit of smoking than children whose parents are non-smokers.

**(ii) High Blook Pressure**

High blood pressure cannot be cured but it can be controlled by changes in lifestyle and if necessary by medication. Some of the ways are:

1. **By maintaining a desirable body weight.** Weight control is an important factor in preventing and controlling high blood pressure.
2. **Reducing sodium intake.** The sodium intake should be 2400 mg or less per day. This is equivalent to about 1.2 teaspoons of salt. In most of the cases, the high blood pressure reduces by reducing the intake of salt. In extreme cases of acute high blood pressure, doctors recommend a salt free diet by replacing sodium salt (sodium chloride) by potassium salt. Potassium chloride is also helpful in reducing high blood pressure.
3. **Reducing consumption of alcoholic beverages.** The daily alcohol intake should not be more than

2 ounce (60 ml) of 100 proof whiskey or its equivalent.

4. **Regular exercises.** The high blood pressure can be decreased or controlled by regular exercising.

**(iii) Cholesterol level**

The cholesterol levels can be kept at the optimum permissible level by taking diet low in fat (especially saturated fat), rich in dietary fibre (rice, corn, apples, dried beans etc.), low in cholesterol (meats, diary products and oils). Moderate drinking, exercising and quitting smoking can also control cholesterol levels.

**(iv) Diabetes**

Like high blood pressure, diabetes cannot be cured but it can be controlled by changes in life-style and if necessary by medication.

**(v) Obesity**

People who are obese are more prone to high blood pressure, diabetes and high cholesterol level leading to heart diseases. Obesity or excess body weight can be controlled by proper diet and exercise.

**(vi) Physical inactivity**

Physical inactivity is a risk factor for coronary heart disease. Becoming active is very important for preserving and/or improving health. Physical activity is indispensable for longevity and for achieving cardiovascular fitness. Some important benefits of regular exercise are:

- Reduction in death rate from all causes.
- Reduction in risk for heart attack and strokes

- Increase in levels of HDL (good) cholesterol and decrease of levels of LDL (bad) cholesterol.
- Lowering blood pressure.
- Lowering triglyceride level.
- Prevention of diabetes.
- Managing stress.

Before starting regular exercises consult your doctor, especially if you are suffering from any cardiovascular disease.

**(vii) Exercise**

Exercise is very important for physical fitness, which, in turn, helps to keep the heart healthy, thereby reducing or lowering the risk (like increasing the level of HDL (good) cholesterol, lowering triglyceride level, lowering blood pressure and prevention of diabetes) of heart attack and stroke.

The quality of life improves considerably if exercise is made a part of life.

**(viii) Nutrition**

The body needs nutrients to function properly (whether in motion or at rest). The common nutrients needed by the body are carbohydrates, proteins, fats, vitamin and minerals. Strictly speaking, water is not a nutrient but is essential for the body to function properly. Good eating habits can significatly decrease the risk of heart disease, stroke, high blood pressure, diabetes and some types of cancer. Most of the nutrients are provided by the food we consume. The common foods are bread, cereal, rice and pasta, fruits, vegetables, meat, poultry, fish, dry beans, eggs and nuts, milk, yogurt and cheese, fats, oils and sweets. The last three should be used very sparingly.

The food consumed must contain various vitamins (which are required to perform specific functions and to- regulate body's metabolism). It has been found that some vitamins like vitamin A, C and E prevent heart disease. Besides vitamins the food also must supply the essential mineral. The tables 7.1, 7.2 and 7.3 given below the vitamins, and minerals along with their source and functions:

**Table 7.1. Vitamins and their functions**

| Vitamin | Source | Function/Essential for |
|---|---|---|
| Vitamin A1 (and beta carotene)[1] | Fish liver oils, liver, butter, margarine, milk and cheese, beta carotene found in carrots, sweet potatoes, pumpkins, green leafy vegetables and fruits (cantaloupe, peaches, broccoli, mustard green and spinach) | Healthy skin, strong teeth and bones in children. Maintaining resistance to infection, normal vision. important role in hormone development and cell structure. Retard oxidation of LDL (bad) cholesterol and so reduces the chances of heart attack. |
| Vitamin B-1 (thiamine) | Whole grain, brown rice, beans, peas, seeds, nuts. | Normal function of nervous system. Helps in metabolism of carbohydrates, digestion and appetite. |
| Vitamin B-2 (riboflavi-n) | Meat, fish, eggs, milk, green vegetables (broccoli, turnip green, asparagus, spinach) | Normal growth Formation of some enzymes. Prevention of sores of mouth and tongue. |
| Vitamin B-3 (pantothi-nic acid) | Fish, poultry, lean meats, whole grains | Control activities of enzymes in metabolism of fats and carbohydrates. Production of sex hormones. Healthy skins. Function of nervous system and digestive system. |

| | | |
|---|---|---|
| Vitamin B-4[2] (niacin or nicotinic acid) | Meat, fish, chicken, potato, whole grains, ground nuts, tomato, green vegetables | Essential for cell metabolism and absorption of carbohydrates. Helps maintain healthy skin. |
| Vitamin B-6 (Pyridoxi-ne) | Meat, whole grains, wheat germ yeast. | Manufacture of haemoglobin. Metabolism of amino acids. |
| Vitamin B-12 (cyanoco-balamin) | Fish, dairy products, meat, eggs. | Function of nervous system, development of red blood cells. Production of genetic material in cells. |
| Biotin (Vitamin H) | Nuts, whole grains, vegetables, fruits, milk, yeast, meat | Use of carbohydrates and folic acid in the body. |
| Folic Acid[3] (Vitamin M) | Green leafy vegetables, orange, beans, peas, rice, eggs, liver | Activities of certain enzymes needed to break down fatty acids. |
| Vitamin C[4] (ascorbic acid) | Citrus and other fresh fruits and vegetables like broccoli, cabbage, potatoes and pepper | Growth, reproduction, production of red blood cells in the body. Important in metabolic process in the body. |
| Vitamin D (calciferol) | Fish, liver, eggs, fortified milk. | Good for skin, bones, teeth, gums, ligaments. Provides immunity to disease. Increase body ability to absorb iron from food. Promotes wound healing and some enzymes reaction. Reduces severity of cold virus. Lower risk of cancers of stomach and esophagus. |
| Vitamin E[5] (tocopher-ol) | Whole grains, vegetables oils, green leafy vegetables, eggs | Strong bones, regulates absorption of calcium and phosphorous from digestive tract. |
| Vitamin K (phyllo quinone) | Green leafy vegetables, dairy products | Formation of red blood cells. Some neuro logic functions. Protection against pollutants. Blood clotting. |

## Notes

1. Prolonged intake of high doses of vitamin A (greater than 50,000 international units) can be toxic and may cause headaches, vomiting, bone abnormalities and liver damage.
2. Niacin or nicotinic acid is considered to lower high blood pressure. It is also very effective in lowering LDL (bad) cholesterol levels and triglycerides, and raising HDL (good) cholesterol levels. Due to its bad side effects, it should be used on advice of a doctor.
3. High Folic acid levels may decrease the absorption of zinc and may mask pernicious anemia. It should be taken under guidance of a physician.
4. Some experts recommend high doses of vitamins C (1000 mg per day) to help lower the blood pressure and lower LDL (bad) cholesterol levels. However higher doses of Vitamin C taken over long periods of time can be dangerous to some people. Vitamin C supplements should be taken under doctor's advice.
5. Vitamin E prevents heart disease, cancer and Parkinson's disease. It prevents the oxidation of LDL (bad) cholesterol and also the heart disease.

## Table 7.2. Minerals, their source and uses

| Minerals | Source | Necessary for |
|---|---|---|
| Calcium | Green leafy vegetables. Dairy products, nuts, legumes | Healthy bones and teeth. Muscles and nerve functions. Blood clotting. Insulin secretion. Enzyme regulation, Production of energy, immunity. |
| Chlorine | Table salt | Maintaining body's fluid and electrolyte balance, digestive juices. |
| Magnesium | Whole grain cereals legumes, many fruits and green vegetables, fish, meat, dairy products | Regulating the conversion of carbohydrates into energy. Formation of hormones and enzymes that regulate various body process. Synthesis of nucleic acid and protein. |

| | | |
|---|---|---|
| Phosphorous | Fish, meat, poultry, vegetable, eggs and dairy products | Strong bones, all cell functions and cell membrane |
| Potassium | Fresh vegetables and fruits | Many major biological processes, muscle contraction nerve conduction. Synthesis of nucleic acid and proteins. |
| Sodium | Table salt | Osmotic equilibrium in tissue |
| Sulphur | Onions, garlic, eggs, meat and dairy products | Sulphur containing amino acid |

## Table 7.3. Trace elements

| Trace elements | Source | Necessary for |
|---|---|---|
| Chromium | Whole grains, spices, meat yeast | Sugar metabolism |
| Copper | Nuts, fruits, shell fish organ meat | Function and synthesis of hemoglobin. Production of collagen, elastin neuro transmitters. |
| Fluorine | Fluorinated water | Binding calcium in bones and teeth |
| Iodine | Iodized salt, sea food | Production of energy (as part of thyroid hormone) |
| Iron | Poultry, fish, meat , organ meat | Synthesis and function of hemoglobin. Enzyme action in energy production. Production of collagen elastin, neuro transmitter. |
| Manganese | Whole grains, nuts | Necessary for optimal health |
| Molybdenum | Whole grains, green leafy vegetables, milk, beans, organ meat | Necessary for optimal health |

| | | |
|---|---|---|
| Selenium | Cabbage, broccoli, celery, onions, garlic, whole grains, yeast, organ meat | Necessary for optimal health |
| Zinc | Whole grains, yeast, fish, meats | Good vision. Immunity and healing. Enzymic activities. |

## Notes

1. Calcium and megnesium help to regulate the heart's rhythm. Abnormal levels of calcium, magnesium and potassium can cause irregular heartbeats, especially in people having heart disease.
2. It has been shown that people who consume less than 300 mg of calcium per day have 2-3 times as great a risk for developing hypertension compared to those who consume 1200 mg per day.
3. A diet deficient in magnesium increase chances of developing high blood pressure, a major risk factor for heart attack and stroke.
4. Eating excess sodium (salt) contributes significantly to high blood pressure. Total intake of sodium should not exceed 2,400 mg a day, which is approximately equal to the amount contained a tablespoon of salt. In case of person suffering from blood pressure the sodium intake has to be considerably reduced or even stopped in extreme cases.
5. Increased iron intake may lead to hemochromatosis, a disease of iron metabolism. It left untreated, it can lead to cardiac disease. Cirrhosis, diabetes, arthritis, cancer of liver. Iron supplements should be taken only on advice of physician.
6. Function of selenium is not entirely understood.

## Guidelines for healthy eating habits

The body needs about 50 different nutrients. The following suggestions will help you in daily eating habits.

1. Eat a variety of foods every day for getting different nutrients.
2. On the basis of your healthy weight eat the right amount. Do not eat more than you need to maintain your healthy weight.

3. Intake of added sugar should not be more than 10% of the total daily calories (eat about 6 tablespoon of sugar for about 1600 calories intake).
4. Intake of complex carbohydrates should be 50% or more of your daily calories.
5. Intake of dietary fibers should be 20-25 grams daily for both soluble and insoluble fibers.
6. Intake of only 0.75 gram of proteins per kilogram of body weight per day.
7. Consumption of fats should not exceed 30% of your total daily calories. For example, if you consume a daily diet of 2000 calories (or 2500 calories), your fat intake for the day should be no more than 65 grams (or 80 grams) (each gram of fat provides 9 calories). Also limit consumption of saturated fats to no more than 10% of total calories (20 grams of fat in a 2000 calories in one day diet).
8. As far as possible use mono unsaturated fats.
9. Limit your consumption of cholesterol to about 300 milligram daily (an egg has 213 milligram of cholesterol).
10. Intake of proteins should be 8-12% of your total daily calories. On an average an adult needs 50-55 grams of proteins per day.
11. Consumption of sodium should be limited to 2400 millligrams (about 1 table spoon of salt per day).
12. People taking vegetarian diet have much less risk for getting cancer.

### 7.4 Diabetes

People suffer from diabetes mellitus or diabetes when the pancreas fail to secrete enough hormone called insulin or when the body loses some of its ability to use insulin. Insulin controls the amout of sugar (or glucose) in the blood. It is also needed to transfer glucose from the blood stream to the cells. In the later situation, the cells are damaged by being starved of the nutrients. Since the cells cannot absorb glucose, its concentration in blood increases. The excess of glucose so accumulated in the blood passes into the urine. The same situation arises in case the pancreas is not able to make the required amout of insulin.

**Symptoms of diabetes**

The common noticeable symptoms of diabetes are greater frequency and volume of urination, feeling thirsty, loosing weight (despite increased appetite), and fatigue. Some of the warning symptoms include blurred vision, numbness in the hands and feet.

It should be understood that diabetes is a chronic illness. It will not disappear and cannot be cured. However, it can be controlled either by modifying the life-style and /or by medication.

In a large number of cases, people do not even realise that they are diabetic. This is because early symptoms may be slight. Even at this level, diabetes is serious. If untreated, diabetes may cause long term damage to the heart, eyes, kidneys and nerves. Diabetics have an increased risk of developing coronary artery disease and suffering a stroke and heart attack. In view of this, it is extremely important to find out by regualar checks whether a person is suffering from diabetes. If detected early, it can be effectively managed. However, if allowed to progress, diabetics can be fatal. Hence, early detection of diabetes is of paramount importance. It can be controlled by proper diet, exercise, stresss management and proper medication.

Everyone is prone to diabetes particularly who has a family history of diabetes and is obese is especially at risk. Damage to pancreas (which are responsible for the production of insulin) either by measles or mumps can also lead to diabetes. It should be understood that by eating or consuming too much sugar, one does not get diabetes. However, a diabetic person must decrease the intake of sugar. Diabetes is more frequent in women than man. Older adults are more susceptible to diabetes.

## Types of Diabetes

There are two types of diabetes:

1. Insulin dependent diabetes (juvenile diabetes) (Type-I). It is caused by severe insulin deficiency, which results from problems with the insulin producing cells in the pancreas. Peak age of onset is 12 years, although it can develop at any stage and insulin must be administered to sustain life. However, life span of people suffering from Type I diabetes is much smaller.

2. Non-insulin dependent diabetes (Type II diabetes). It usually occurs in people over 40 or who become resistant to the insulin produced in their systems. Obese persons are at greater risk for this kind of diabetes. It is found that most of the people who have diabetes belong to Type II diabetes.

## Prevention (or Management) of Diabetes

Following are given some of the guidelines (suggestions) for preventing Diabetes:

### (i) Diet

The diet of a diabetic should be very low in fat and sugar. Normally, in a typical meal, 50-60% of the calories you consume should come from complex carbohydrates, as found in whole-grain breads, cereals, fruits and vegetables. Less than 20% of the calories consumed should come from proteins and less than 30% from fat. It is essential to reduce fat intake because high concentration of fat in the bloodstream can reduce body's ability to use insulin. Simple sugar as found in table sugar, syrup, processed foods, candies, cookies and soft drinks should be avoided.

It is important that a diabetic should drink about 2.5-3 litres of water daily. An ideal diet of diabetic should be rich in vitamin B-6, vitamin B-12, thiamine and magnesium. Whole grain bread, cereals, dried beans, peas and other legumes are good sources for thiamine, magnesium and vitamin B-6. Lean meat is rich in thiamine and vitamins B-6 and B-12. Milk products and eggs are also sources of vitamin B-12.

### (ii) Exercise

In case of diabetics, exercise improves blood circulation throughout the body. This is especially important since diabetes can cause decrease in blood circulation, especially in arms, legs and feet often lead to complications. Exercise decreases the concentration of sugar (glucose) in the blood making the cells in the body more sensitive to insulin.

### (iii) Stress Management

Stress increases the levels of glucose and blood pressure, both harmful for diabetes. It is advisable to take special care to remove stress. Regular exercise keeps your blood pressure and blood sugar levels under control.

Though diabetes is a chronic illness, yet one should learn to live a reasonably healthy life with it. At times, it seems difficult to manage diabetes, especially if you look at it as a life time concern. However, you can cope with it by following a healthy routine. Avoid worrying about it and make best use of the circumstances in which you are placed.

## 7.5 Depression

Depression if not checked in time, makes one feel older than one actually is. There can be may reasons for setting in of depression. Some of the reasons are:

- Pressure of work in the office
- Death in the family
- Not getting along with spouce
- Children leaving home
- Retirement from services
- For women, a important potential trigger for depression is the experience of menopause—the feeling a woman gets that she is not as young as she used to be.

### Effects of Depression

- Depression can turn into an event in which youthfullnesss, vitality and health are lost.
- People having depression are four times more likely to have heart attacks than those who are not depressed.
- Episode of depression can lead to high blood pressure.

- For women, depression may increase chances of developing osteoporosis.

**Prevention or dealing with depresion**

It is well known that a number of drugs are available to fight depression. It is important to know that the body has its own defenses. Chemicals which are responsible for altering of the mood are constantly flowing through the body; these in turn effect emotions and health. During exercise, for instance, the brain start producing endorphins, neurotransmitters that can improve mood and even remove pain. In fact exercise can do what the antidepressants do. Thus, exercise programme helps to ward off depression. Following are given some other procedures which prevent depression.

- Do what you enjoy. Any thing that is fun for you or you enjoy doing (e.g., walking, biking, rowing, swimming, etc.) will keep the depression at bay.
- The easiest is walking. In fact, walking comes to the resque in case of depression.
- Never dewel on the fact that you are depressed, since it is a vicious cycle. The more you think about being depressed, the more depressed you get.
- Retire is a single biggest example which causes depression. The main problem is that people who are very busy find it difficult to pass time after retirement. After retirement, people are virtually cut off from their colleague and other activities. One should plan couple of years before retirement as the how one will keep busy doing useful work "Empty mind is a devils workshop" and so remaining idle invites depression.

- **Group sports.** These give you the benefit of exercise and also being in the company of others.
- **Yoga classes.** These also give you the benefit of exercise and also bring in the company of others.
- **Getting a pet.** Pet is a very good sincere companion and will keep you busy.
- Avoid drugs, alcohol and caffeine.

## 7.6 Constipation

It is directly related to digestive system. The muscles of the intestines gradually loses tone and get weaker as one ages. Also eating too much fat and not getting enough dietary fibre adds to the problem. The digestive system's efficiency is reduced or slowed down in the sixtees; the stomach begins to secrete lower than normal amounts of stomach begin to secrete lower than normal amouts of stomach acid, which is responsible for stomach pain. Besides, it can also inhibit body's absorption capacity of calcium and iron, causing anemia and osteoporosis.

It should be understood that normally it is said that a person is constipated if he/she is not regular in bowel movement. However, it is known that for some people it is normal for going once in three days and for others it is normal going three times a day. So constipation varies from person to person and it is for him or her to define what is normal for him/her. However, if bowel movement is possible only by straining, it can lead to hemorrhoids– a condition that sets in when veins around the rectum swell under pressure and turn painful.

It is known that constipation can be treated by using lexatives. Using lexatives only occasionally it is possible to relieve temporary constipation. But use of lexdatives once a week or more can make constipation worse. In such cases, the body's natural mechanism starts to depend on lexative for prompt bowel movement. This is, no doubt is not good for the system. Thus, though constipation can be treated, why not prevent them-which is possible by making a few changes in diet and life-style.

### Prevention of Constipation

Constipation can be prevented or in other words, digestion can be improved by the suggestions/ guidelines:

(i) **Diet**

One should consume more fibre, which improves muscle function in the colon by making the stool bigger and stretching the intestinal muscles which makes them contract better. One should consume 20-30 grams of fibre per day to maintain a healthy digestive track and to avoid constipation. Following foods are recommended for getting fibre:

- Wheat given
- Squash (mashed)
- whole wheat bread
- backed eyed peas, cooked
- kidney beans, cooked
- spinach, cooked
- broccolli, boiled
- sweet potato, baked

**(ii) Drink plenty of water**

One should drink two litres of water per day. In fact, the combination of water and fiber increase the bulk of the stool.

(iii) **Exercise Programme**

Among the exercises that improve digestion are walking, swimming programme for 30 minutes daily is the best for good results.

(iv) **Avoid Peppers**

Both red and green peppers contain 'capsaium', a chemical, which make the bowel movements irritable.

(v) **Avoid Fried Food**

(vi) **Relaxing**

(vii) **Reduce Fat in you diet**

(viii) **Keep body weight in control.**

# 8

# The Golden Procedure for Delaying the Onset of Aging

## 8.1 Naturopathy

According to Naturopaths, falling sick over and over again leads to premature aging. In fact, a person falls sick when the defense of his system or body goes down. This defense system is described as the vital force. The modern physicians attribute this so called vital force to the immune system. In order to live a healthy life, free of any sickness one should follow the simple rules or the laws of nature as given below:

**(i) Sound sleep:**

One gets sound sleep, if one is completely relaxed. It is very helpful to inhale deeply a few times before going off to sleep. In case there is difficulty to get sound sleep one should practice meditation. Under no circumstances tranquilizers should be taken.

**(ii) Living in fresh air:**

The oxygen present in air helps the lungs to clean the blood of carbon dioxide. The house should be well ventilated so that fresh air comes in contact with the body all the time. Deep breathing helps the lungs to take in more oxygen and also get rid of carbon dioxide in the blood. Also living in air-conditioned houses and or working in air-conditioned offices is not healthy. In such an event, the air in the house/office should be replaced by outside fresh air.

**(iii) Sunlight:**

It is essential for the body. Like sleep, it helps to restore one's vital force and also helps the body to synthesize Vitamin D, which is essential for a healthy body.

**(iv) Water:**

It is essential for sustaining life and health. Water should be fresh and should be untreated. The best is to consume plenty of vegetables and fruits as these supply the best quality of water. It is advisable to drink water, which has been exposed to sunlight. A daily cold-water bath is very helpful for delaying the onset of aging. When the skin is cooled by cold water, blood rushes to warm it up. The circulation of blood is activated and the blood is also cleansed of many impurities. A slowed down circulation is a prelude to old age. A cold bath is therefore, instrumental in keeping us young.

**(v) Diet:**

A greater part of the diet should comprise of fruits and vegetables and should be taken raw if possible. If cooked, vegetables should be lightly cooked or steam cooked.

**(vi) Life-style:**

Life should be clean, free from any addiction of any type. Over indulgence in any activity reduces the vital force. Life should be free of tension and stress. Exercise helps us stay healthy.

## 8.2 Meditation

Meditation is an Indian ancient discipline. It involves contemplation while focusing one's mind on a thought or an object. It is a practice that enables us to understand every thing in life clearly. It is a type of mental exercise. It is an awakening state of consciousness. Some of the benefits of meditation are:

- It is a very powerful mental and nerve tonic.
- It removes all pain suffering and sorrows.
- During meditation, there is a reduction of the activity in the nervous system.
- It has a significant effect on the way the brain works.
- The quality of sleep improves when meditation is practiced regularly.
- It develops an individual's will power, the power of decision.
- It helps to work with concentration.
- The most important effect of meditation is that it reduces stress. We know that stress is one factor responsible for premature aging.
- Meditation helps to lead a long and happy life.

Posture is very important in meditation. A number of postures can be used. A simple and easy posture involves sitting across cross-legged with both feet on the floor. The back should be straight but not tensed and stomach muscles relaxed. With the muscles of the lower back bearing the weight of the body and with the head, neck and trunk in line, the center of gravity passes from the back of the spine right through the top of the head. The hands can either rest lightly on the knees or be held in the lap, either one on top of the other or clasped lightly.

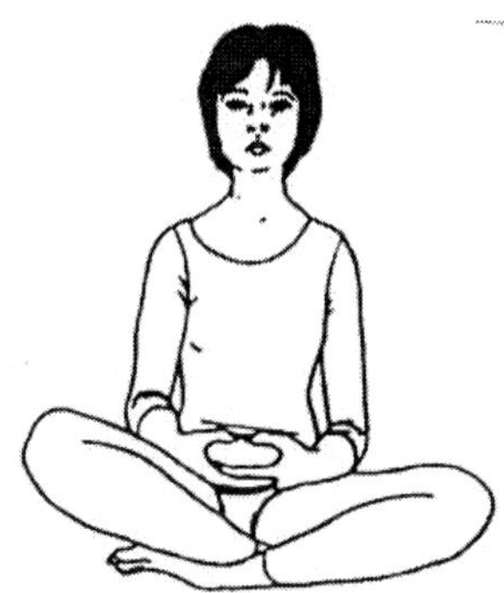

**Fig. 8.1. The easy posture**

Another easy posture is called shavasana or the corpse position. Lie flat on the floor on a carpet, blanket or hard mattress. Part the legs a little and let the feet flop at the sides. The arms should be slightly away from the body, hands on the floor and palms up.

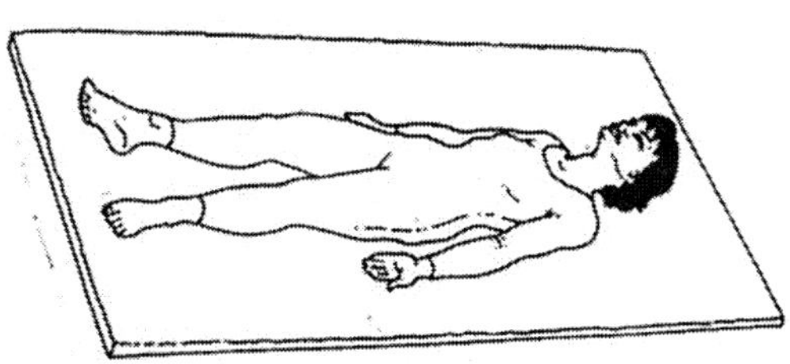

**Fig. 8.2. Lying flat**

There are many different methods of meditation. One can start the program of meditation with the basic meditation called breath counting. It is basically to teach and practice the ability to do one thing at a time. It looks simple. In fact, it is very hard and requires a great deal of practice and if done properly has definite positive psychological and physiological effects. Follow the following steps:

*(i)* Place yourself in a comfortable position so that one gets few distracting signals from the body. This can be done lying on the floor, sitting or standing depending on an individual's convenience.

*(ii)* Now count silently each time you break out, so count 1 for the first breath, 2 for the second, 3 for the third and 4 for the fourth breath. And then start again with one.

*(iii)* Keep repeating the above procedure until 15 minutes. You can find the time either by facing the clock where you can see it without moving your head. Alternatively, set a 15-minute alarm.

Note: A number of feelings will come to your mind. No matter what other thoughts, feelings or perceptions come during 15 minutes, your task is simply to do the counting. Let the thoughts and feelings come and pass without your getting involved with these. Just keep watching them and concentrating on your breaths. Conscious of any thing else during this period is wandering away from the task. Normally one does not do well at all, to be able to succeed for more than couple of seconds at a time in being aware only of your counting. This takes long practice.

There are a number of variations of the above breath counting meditation. Some people prefer to count up to 10 and keep repeating. Still another variation is to keep on counting up to 15 minutes, to as high as you can go. In the latter method it is very difficult to avoid self-competition. Count of 4 seems to be the best available course.

It should be noted that breathing in this way can produce dizziness and nausea and should not be practiced by pregnant women, anyone with hyper or hypo tension or with lung problems. It is best learned from a teacher than from the pages of this writing.

A technique called bellows breathing or bhastrika pranayam, is recommended by experts on meditation to quieten the mind before proper meditation begins. The procedure involves breathing in and out rapidly by forcing abdominal muscles to expand and contract rapidly. It takes some practice to breathe properly in this way. It should be not attempted until three hours after eating, and should eat nothing for at least half an hour afterwards.

Many meditators use a mantra, a word or a phrase repeated again and again either out loud or in mind.

Any physical discomfort makes meditation difficult. The discomfort could be a worry or unresolved problem or something that has made you angry. One way to get rid of physical tension is to focus attention on each part of the body for a moment tensed and then relax it slowly. Deep slow breathing can also help. Concentrate as hard as you can and as you breath out, try to imagine the pain or tension evaporating.

Besides the technique for meditation, a number of other techniques are also used. For this, consult a meditation teacher. In fact all meditations should be done and practiced in the correct way in the presence of a meditation teacher.

The benefits of meditation, if done on a routine basis are amazing. This is one of the best ways to make life free of worries and tensions. This in turn slows down aging and helps us live a long and healthy life.

# 9

# CONCLUSION

There is no single pill, vitamin, mineral, herb, food or other substances known to ward off aging. One has to raise levels of many antioxidants to best deter aging against free radical damage and other contributors of aging. The most important is the antioxidant status. Most of us (healthy adults) need the following supplements to stop or delay aging according to latest knowledge based on research.

- Multivitamin- mineral tablet with 100% of RDA for most vitamins, minerals and trace elements
- Vitamin E (100-400 iu)
- Vitamin C (500-1500 mg)
- Beta-carotene (10-15 mg)
- Chromium (200 micrograms)
- Calcium (500-1500 mg)
- Zinc (15-30 mg)
- Selenium (15-200 micrograms)
- Magnesium (200-300 mg)
- Coenzyme Q –10 (30 mg)

Note:

1. One can usually get enough anti-aging B Vitamins, including folic acid in a multivitamin-mineral pill. However, one may need separate B vitamin tablets in higher doses for specific reasons.

2. The doses given are in different ranges and how much one needs, depends on individual circumstances.
3. "More is always good" is not necessarily true, since high doses can be toxic and detrimental.
4. High doses should be taken only in consultation with a physician.
5. Supplements can interact with other medications to produce adverse affects. Therefore a doctor should be consulted.

In addition to the above, other anti-aging daily supplements should be taken (given below) if one is older or have symptoms of any specific age related diseases or if one is about 45 years old.

- B Vitamins
  - B12 – 1000 micrograms
  - B 6 – 50 mg
  - Folic Acid – 1000 micrograms
- Gingko – 40 mg tablet (three daily)
- Glutathione – 100 mg
- Glutamine 2000-8000 mg
- Fish oil concentrate in capsules–1000 mg of a combination of DHA and EPA fatty acids
- Garlic supplements—If one does not eat garlic, take 6 capsules of garlic powder.
- L-carnitite—1000-2000 mg (if an individual has angina, heart arrhyttmias or mild signs of heart failure.

One should take anti-aging diet consisting of

- Fruits and vegetables at least 5 servings a day.
- Eat fish, 2-3 times a week.
- Drink tea.
- Soybean foods, 2-3 times a day.

- Restrict calories to maintain normal weight.
- Restrict the wrong or bad fats. Use olive oil, canola oil and other mono saturated oils like macadamia nut oil.
- Restrict or avoid meat.
- Drink alcohol in moderation. Wine is useful (particularly red wine)
- Curb sweets.
- Eat garlic.

Finally, there are no final and complete answers on postponing aging as of today. The data given above is on the basis of correct but incomplete research.

# Notes:

# Notes:

## Notes: